The Kitchen Table Book ③

Even More Kitchen Secrets, Forgotten Cures, and Pantry Potions for Every Health and Household Problem

Publisher's Note

This book is intended for general information only. It does not constitute medical, legal, or financial advice or practice. The editors of FC&A have taken careful measures to ensure the accuracy and usefulness of the information in this book. While every attempt has been made to ensure accuracy, errors may occur. Some websites, addresses, and telephone numbers may have changed since printing. We cannot guarantee the safety or effectiveness of any advice or treatments mentioned. Readers are urged to consult with their professional financial advisors, lawyers, and health care professionals before making any changes.

Any health information in this book is for information only and is not intended to be a medical guide for self-treatment. It does not constitute medical advice and should not be construed as such or used in place of your doctor's medical advice. Readers are urged to consult with their health care professionals before undertaking therapies suggested by the information in this book, keeping in mind that errors in the text may occur as in all publications and that new findings may supersede older information.

The publisher and editors disclaim all liability (including any injuries, damages, or losses) resulting from the use of the information in this book.

Dear friend, I pray that you may enjoy good health and that all may go well with you, even as your soul is getting along well.
— *3 John 1:2 (NIV)*

Table of Contents

Pantry staples

Aloe vera 2

Aspirin 7

Baking soda 10

    A closer look: Emergency substitutions 18

Chocolate 19

Honey 25

    A closer look: Sugar and other sweeteners 29

Nutritional yeast 31

Olive oil 35

Vinegar 43

Vegetables

Beets 52

Broccoli 55

Cabbage 60

Cauliflower 63

Eggplant 67

Garlic 70

A closer look: Juicing 76

Greens 78

Onions 86

Peppers 90

A closer look: Going organic 97

Potatoes 98

Tomatoes 103

Fruits

Apples 110

Apricots 115

Avocados 119

Bananas 125

Berries 129

A closer look: Storing produce 136

Cherries 137

Citrus 142

Figs 149

A closer look: Exotic fruits 152

Grapes 154

Melons 159

Prunes 164

Whole grains

Barley 168

Brown rice 173

Oats 176

Popcorn 182

Quinoa 185

A closer look: Ancient grains 191

Sorghum 193

Wheat bran 197

A closer look: Best breads 200

Legumes

Beans 202

A closer look: Bean swaps 208

Chickpeas 209

Lentils 214

A closer look: Slow cookers 219

Peanuts 220

Soybeans 224

Fermented foods

Kefir 230

    A closer look: Prebiotics 233

Kimchi 234

Kombucha 238

Miso 241

Sauerkraut 245

    A closer look: Fermentation and probiotics 250

Yogurt 251

Nuts & Seeds

Chia seeds 258

Fennel seeds 261

Flaxseeds 263

Pecans 267

Sesame seeds 271

Walnuts 274

Seafood

Oysters 280

Salmon 284

A closer look: Grilling and marinating 292

Sardines 294

Beverages

Coffee 300

Plant milks 306

Skim milk 314

Tea 318

Water 325

Spices & herbs

Anise 334

Cinnamon 336

Cloves 340

A closer look: Low-salt diet 343

Ginseng 345

Rosemary 348

Sage 352

Turmeric 355

Index
Index 361

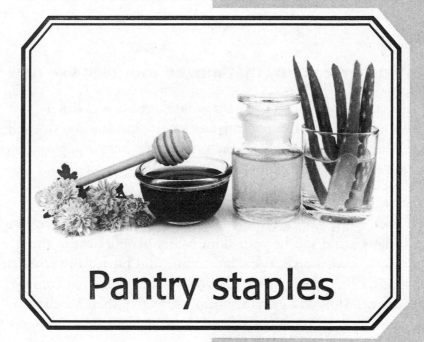

Pantry staples

Aloe vera

An ancient remedy that makes your skin like new

You've heard of Queen Cleopatra's intelligence and beauty, but did you know you can tap into her smart skin routine yourself? She's said to have used aloe vera gel to keep her royal glow. Chances are, she also knew these skin-saving secrets about aloe.

Bandage up burns with aloe. Whether you've scorched yourself with a hot pan or sat in the bright light of the sun too long, this plant could soothe your skin. Many people turn to the antibiotic cream silver sulfadiazine for mild burns. But research has found that aloe vera cream works better than that common treatment. Aloe vera gel is also more effective than Vaseline gauze. It may help lower recovery time, prevent infection, and reduce redness and itchiness.

Although its cooling effect is one reason it's useful for burns, aloe's wound-healing power largely stems from its antioxidant and anti-inflammatory properties. No surprise that it could improve other skin injuries, too, like pressure sores and ulcers.

The skinny on moisturizing your skin. Aloe grows comfortably in the dry desert, but it's excellent at keeping your skin hydrated. That's at least partially because of special long chains of sugar molecules called mucopolysaccharides. They help bind moisture to your skin.

Aloe can also help soften your skin and keep it healthy. That's important because your skin is a protective barrier against things like trauma and temperature changes.

Be careful not to overuse aloe vera, though. This plant also contains enzymes that act as an exfoliator. That can make it useful for skin smoothing, but too much can circle back around to drying out your skin. So don't slather it on more than three times daily.

You can scoop the aloe gel from the plant yourself and apply it to your skin. Or just purchase an over-the-counter gel or lotion containing aloe.

 Watch out

First things first. Aloe vera gel is the thick, clear pulp in the middle of the leaf that has a tender consistency similar to extra-firm jelly. To get to it, you'll have to go through two plant layers.

Don't eat the outer skin or the sappy coating just under the skin. The aloin found in this yellow sap, called the latex layer, is a strong laxative and can cause diarrhea and stomach cramps.

Fortunately, it's easy to remove those pesky outer layers. After carefully washing the leaves, cut off their sharp tips and spiky sides. Cut the leaves down into manageable rectangles, and let them soften in a bowl of water for 10 to 20 minutes. Then use a sharp knife to slice open the leaves and remove the clear gel from the outer layers. Some of the yellow aloin may be left on it, so rinse the gel in water again, and then you're good to go.

Jazz up your health with aloe juice

Like your body, aloe vera is mostly water. All that liquid makes this succulent a great option for juice, which you can buy at the store or make at home by blending the gel with water. What's more, aloe juice can flood your body with healthful benefits.

Take a sip to soothe internal burning. The fight against heart-burn and acid reflux doesn't have to be all antacids from a bottle. You may be able to reduce your symptoms with the help of aloe vera. This plant can be soothing to your digestive tract, and the benefits extend to the burning irritation you may get with reflux.

New research tackles thyroid troubles. Aloe vera has been harnessed as a remedy for thousands of years. Now a study fresh off the presses suggests it may have another calling — a treatment for improving thyroid function.

A small study recruited a group of women with Hashimoto's thyroiditis-related hypothyroidism. This condition, caused by an autoimmune disease, happens when the thyroid gland doesn't produce enough hormones. For nine months, the participants drank just over 1.5 ounces of aloe juice each day.

The researchers found that this reduced thyroid inflammation and improved thyroid function and hormone production. More research is needed, but these results show promise.

Grab the reins on your blood sugar. Aloe is a pretty unassuming plant, so you might never guess just glancing at it that it could help you take control of your diabetes. But some research suggests that it may do just that.

Studies of aloe have followed its effect on both prediabetes and type 2 diabetes, both of which feature insulin resistance, meaning your body isn't using insulin properly to balance the amount of sugar in your blood. Research indicates that aloe may help with this by lowering blood sugar and improving your body's insulin response.

Keep this in mind when shopping

You can find aloe juice at your local grocery store, but don't buy just any old bottle.

Look into the reputation of the company and read the label for clues about manufacturing. For example, whole leaf aloe must be filtered to remove the latex, which could affect quality if not done properly. Inner leaf aloe can bypass this step but is often more expensive.

You should also keep a close eye on the percentage of aloe. You want it to be as close to 100% as possible. Since you're looking for health benefits, try to keep the sugar content down, too. You may find aloe mixed with other drinks, like teas or fruit juices, but this isn't the same as pure aloe juice and will likely have few active ingredients that will actually benefit your health.

Check with your doctor before adding aloe into your diet, and start at just 1 ounce of juice a day to see how your body responds.

The plant pathway to a better night

You've got your nighttime routine down pat. But before lights out, incorporate some aloe into your evening habits for a little positive push.

Tighten up dental defenses. You know to look for the American Dental Association's seal of approval for fluoride in your toothpaste, but have you ever bought a tube of aloe vera tooth gel? You might want to try it out.

Some research suggests that aloe vera tooth gel fights off bad bacteria in your mouth that causes cavities. As an added bonus, it's especially great if you have sensitive teeth because this gel is less abrasive than toothpaste.

Dead set on your favorite toothpaste? No worries. Add aloe vera to your dental care as a mouthwash. You can swish it to fight gingivitis, a form of gum disease that can lead to infection.

Air out a bad sleep cycle. Aloe is welcome at slumber time. This low-maintenance potted plant could improve your sleep just by sitting in your room with you.

Research suggests that high oxygen levels might help you achieve deeper, more restful sleep. While indoor foliage won't offer the same levels used in the study, aloe — like other plants — is an expert at absorbing carbon dioxide and releasing oxygen.

NASA has researched the benefits of greenery, too. It found that aloe is among the plants that can filter out some harmful chemicals from the air. Other space data suggests that plants can improve your physical and mental health, including your sleep. This study didn't include aloe, but does speculate that the green color of the plants may have been one of the positive influences.

 Kitchen hacks

Don't let the unusual gooey-firm texture of aloe vera gel scare you off from eating it. You can try it plain, but if you're feeling adventurous or want to disguise the slightly bitter plant-like taste, add it as an ingredient to your recipes. See if any of these pique your fancy.

- Poach the gel over low heat with some citrus juice and sugar. The resulting jello-like treat can become topping for your yogurt or dessert.

- Hide the flavor of aloe gel by blending it into a tasty fruit smoothie.

- Add slices of aloe gel to a stew or soup for some texture.

- Find your favorite ceviche recipe and cube some aloe gel to join the mix.

Aspirin

Should you take an aspirin a day? When to start or skip this popular treatment

It used to be a common practice to pop a baby aspirin every day to keep your heart healthy. After all, experts thought low doses of these cheap pills were packed with benefits at a minimal risk. But new research is prompting many doctors to change their tune on this treatment.

While the occasional pill to treat a headache or a sore muscle doesn't carry too much risk to most people, newer studies have shown that regular, daily aspirin use could have serious side effects.

In a recent review of research, the U.S. Preventive Services Task Force found that people who took aspirin every day or every other day increased their risk of major intestinal bleeding by 58% compared to people who didn't take aspirin. And the risk of hemorrhagic strokes — which are caused by uncontrolled bleeding in the brain — increased by 27%.

So how do you know if aspirin isn't right for you?

- Age. The older you get, the more likely you are to encounter serious bleeding as a result of daily aspirin use. The American College of Cardiology recommends that most people over the age of 70 avoid taking this drug every single day.

- Preexisting conditions and medications. Certain underlying issues, such as diabetes, a history of bleeding in your gastrointestinal tract, or a blood clotting disorder, may increase the likelihood of dangerous side effects from aspirin. Experts also warn that certain medications — like anticoagulants and antidepressants — can cause unsafe interactions with aspirin.

But that doesn't mean aspirin falls short on health benefits. Experts think this medication is still a good way to keep your ticker safe if you're at high risk of heart attack or coronary artery disease. It thins out your blood and prevents platelets from clumping together, which can help keep hazardous blockages from forming in your blood vessels.

Consult your doctor before making any changes to your daily medications. In some cases, they may decide that the heart-healthy benefits of aspirin outweigh the risks. And if you already take this drug every day, suddenly stopping may increase your risk of blood clots and heart attacks.

 Bright idea

In ancient Egypt, physicians used the powdered bark of willow trees to soothe irritated skin. Little did they know that this treatment worked so well because willow bark is loaded with salicylic acid, which is one of the main active ingredients in aspirin.

These days, if you have an inflammatory skin condition like rosacea, psoriasis, or acne, you can make a cheap treatment using aspirin. Start by crushing a few uncoated tablets into a fine powder and stirring them into enough hot water to make a thick paste. Let it cool for a few minutes.

Some people's skin is more sensitive to the ingredients in aspirin, so be sure to do a patch test. Once you know you're in the clear, spread the paste onto itchy, red patches and let it sit for 10 minutes before rinsing off.

A cheap way to keep migraines at bay

Flashing and swirling shapes in your vision, lights that seem far too bright, and sounds that are just too loud — all unwelcome warnings for millions of migraine sufferers. These painful, throbbing headaches often last four hours to three days if left untreated. But new research has found evidence to suggest that quick, cheap relief from migraines may already be hiding in your medicine cabinet.

A new paper published in *The American Journal of Medicine* found that taking high doses of aspirin — between 900 and 1,300 milligrams (mg) — can offer relief from sudden, severe symptoms. And what's even better? This cheap, over-the-counter treatment was just as effective as expensive migraine medications.

The trick is to take about 1,000 mg — or two extra-strength aspirin pills — right when you notice the first signs of a migraine attack. Be on the lookout for a sudden sensitivity to light, sounds, or smells. Also notice if you start to experience nausea or a throbbing or pulsing pain in your head.

If you get frequent migraines, talk to your doctor about taking a baby aspirin every day. The research showed that lower doses of aspirin — think 81 to 325 mg a day — could help prevent recurrent migraines.

Because taking aspirin could have side effects, make sure to clear the dosage with your doctor before you try it out.

If you take an aspirin every day, you may notice that you bruise more easily. Because aspirin keeps blood from clotting, more blood may leak out when the tiny blood vessels under your skin get damaged, causing bruises to form. Fortunately, experts say this typically isn't a sign of a more serious side effect.

Baking soda

Nontoxic cleaning secrets for your whole house

People in the U.S. spend about $170 every year on cleaning supplies. But you don't need to drop hundreds of dollars to make your house shine.

In fact, as long as you're never without five pantry staples, you'll be able to tackle nearly any mess in these key areas of your home. And the best part? It costs less than $10 for the lot of 'em.

Baking soda keeps your kitchen sparkling. A box of baking soda costs just 75 cents. And it will help you clean up greasy, stubborn stains in mere minutes. If you want your kitchen to look so clean that people will think you hired a professional, make sure you always have some on hand.

Simply sprinkle it onto oily pots and pans and let it sit for a few minutes before scrubbing it off. You'll be left with shiny cookware in no time.

And you can even make an all-purpose cleaner with 2 parts baking soda to 1 part water. Use it to scrub dingy grout, grimy sinks, and gunky microwaves and ovens.

Vinegar and rubbing alcohol leave your bathroom spotless. Streaky mirrors? Don't rush out and spend a fortune on glass cleaner when you may already have the solution right in your medicine cabinet. Use a mix of equal parts rubbing alcohol and water to remove soap stains on windows, glass shower doors, and mirrors. Plus polish your stainless steel faucet handles to a shine.

And vinegar can help you scour your bathtub, sink, toilet, and shower. This powerful, natural cleaner attacks mildew, mineral deposit stains, and mold.

All you need to do is spray it on and let it sit for a few minutes before scrubbing it off. For more stain-dissolving action, sprinkle some baking soda on top of the vinegar.

Freshen your bedroom with a cornstarch combo. Your room should be a calming oasis. But how can you kick back and relax if you're constantly surrounded by odors and grime? Fortunately, sprucing up your bedroom is a breeze if you have cornstarch and baking soda handy.

It may sound odd, but the pairing is perfect for brightening your mattress. Next time you wash your sheets, simply sprinkle a mix of baking soda and cornstarch all over your mattress. Let it sit for a few hours and vacuum it up.

The cornstarch will soak up body oils, while baking soda will leave the mattress smelling fresh.

Keep your carpet spick-and-span with liquid detergent. Carpet stains don't need to be a daunting cleaning task if you have the right tools. Good thing your kitchen is already stocked with all you need.

Start by mixing a teaspoon of clear dish soap into a cup of lukewarm water. Dip a clean, white cloth into your mixture and dab it onto carpet stains. Let it soak in for about 15 to 20 minutes before gently scrubbing as needed and blotting up any excess liquid.

If odors are left behind, use baking soda to deodorize the carpet naturally. Sprinkle it on dry carpet, and let it sit for a few hours or overnight before vacuuming thoroughly.

Soda ash: The most powerful cleaner you've never heard of

Sometimes baking soda doesn't have quite enough oomph to tackle every stain and splotch. But you don't need to splash cash on a stronger cleaner. Instead, use your oven to make a powerful degreaser.

Baking soda — also known as sodium bicarbonate — transforms into sodium carbonate when heated. The result? A stronger base, called soda ash or washing soda, that you can use to take on some of your toughest messes.

Line a baking sheet with foil and cover it with baking soda. Bake it in a 350-degree oven for one to two hours. Store it in an airtight container.

Like baking soda, you can mix it with water to make a paste or diluted solution. Just avoid scrubbing it on delicate surfaces. Wear gloves when handling because the powder can cause skin damage and irritation. If you do get it on your skin, thoroughly rinse the area with cool water.

Head-to-toe hygiene: How to care for your body without the steep price tag

Tired of wasting all your cash on beauty supplies? If you want to keep yourself feeling fresh and healthy, you don't have to have deep pockets. A simple, cheap box of baking soda may be all you need.

Get oils and product out of your hair with a scrub. Washing with baking soda may help keep your tresses shiny and soft. Make a paste from a few spoonfuls of baking soda and warm water, rub it into your hair, then rinse. Just don't do this more than once or twice a month. Experts warn that baking soda's high pH can damage your hair and irritate your scalp if you apply it too often.

Make your own deodorant. Because baking soda can neutralize odor-causing bacteria, you can use it to keep your skin smelling fresh and clean. Mix a small amount with water to make a paste, and apply it to your armpits as a low-cost alternative to deodorant. If you're not a fan of the powder residue on your skin, look for commercial deodorants with baking soda in them.

Soothe bug bites, rashes, and itchy skin. Baking soda can help relieve stinging and redness caused by inflammation. Make a paste by mixing 3 parts baking soda with 1 part water, and spread it over bothersome skin. Let it sit for a few minutes before rinsing off.

Banish foot funk. Smelly feet? Dissolve a few spoonfuls of baking soda into a tub of warm water and let your feet soak for about 10 to 15 minutes. To deodorize your shoes, sprinkle a bit of baking soda in them at night and dump it out in the morning.

Clear clogged drains like Roto-Rooter

Chemical clog-busters could damage your pipes and cause massive repair bills if you're not careful. But you can clear plugged up drains with these three ingredients.

Bring a pot of water to a boil and carefully pour half of it down the drain. If you have PVC pipes, let the water cool a bit first so that you don't damage them. Next, add a cup of baking soda and a cup of vinegar, cover your drain, and wait 10 minutes. The bubbling, fizzing reaction that's caused when they mix will help break up the gunk plugging up your pipes. Finally, pour the rest of the water down the drain.

If that doesn't work, dissolve 1 cup of salt and 1 cup of baking soda into 4 cups of boiling or hot water. Pour the mixture down your drain and let it sit overnight before flushing out the drain with hot water.

Bright idea

If you want to extend the life span of your car battery, you'll need to keep it clean. And the best way to do that? Use baking soda to scrub off corrosion and grime.

Start by disconnecting your battery from your car. Make sure your engine is turned off, and use a wrench to remove the negative — or black — wire from the negative battery terminal first. Next remove the positive — or red — cable from the positive terminal.

Here's where things get interesting. Mix 3 tablespoons of baking soda with 3 tablespoons of water to form a thick paste. Use an old toothbrush to apply this paste to the battery terminals, and then scrub it off with a stiff-bristled brush and wipe it clean.

After the battery is dry, add a bit of petroleum jelly to the terminals and reconnect the wires, starting with the red wire so you don't short the battery.

Want whiter teeth? This cheap solution will make your smile sparkle

You know that baking soda can scrub away stains on your countertops and leave you with sparkling pots and pans. But did you know that these incredible cleaning powers aren't only good for household messes?

Dentists have long known that baking soda is a great way to whiten your teeth. But there's even more that it can do. A recent study has found that baking soda may fend off plaque and a form of gum disease called gingivitis.

The study, published in the *American Journal of Dentistry*, compared traditional, fluoride-based toothpaste to ones that were fortified with baking soda.

Researchers instructed participants to brush with one of the toothpastes and evaluated their dental health, including how much plaque they had. At the end of six months, they found that the baking soda toothpastes were better at reducing plaque and gingival inflammation and bleeding.

Want to try it yourself? You can buy toothpastes that already come packed with baking soda. Or simply add a tiny pinch of baking soda to the toothpaste you already have before you brush your teeth.

This surprising remedy may help keep your kidneys in tiptop shape

Waste and toxins can build up in your bloodstream over time. And your body needs a way to filter out everything you don't need in order to stay in fine form. That's where your kidneys come in. These two organs filter out your blood and help keep your body healthy.

But what happens when they stop working? You may need to resort to expensive treatments and procedures — like dialysis — to help your kidneys stop waste from building up in your body. Or you might find relief in your pantry.

Surprisingly, baking soda has shown some promise to help slow the progression of chronic kidney disease. In a study conducted by South Korean researchers, some 70 patients with advanced chronic kidney disease were split into two groups. All of them received standard treatment for the disease, but one group also took baking soda supplements.

At the end of 12 months, the people with stage 4 chronic kidney disease who took baking soda showed a slower rate of kidney decline than people who only received standard medical care. One reason? Experts think that baking soda may reduce the acidity of blood in the body, which helps keep struggling kidneys functioning longer.

People in the study started off by taking about 3 grams — or a little more than half a teaspoon — of baking soda supplements each day, then the researchers adjusted their dose based on their individual needs.

Before you start taking baking soda, talk to your doctor. Because this compound is high in sodium, it could cause problems if you have high blood pressure.

 Kitchen hacks

How old is that box of baking soda sitting in your pantry? And more importantly, is it still good? Baking soda may not come printed with an expiration date on the package. So when you stumble across an old box, chances are you won't actually remember when you bought it.

Fortunately, baking soda can last for 18 months if it's unopened and stored in a cool, dry place. But before you add a dash to your batch of cookies, you might want to test its potency.

All you have to do is simply mix a pinch of it with a bit of vinegar. If it bubbles immediately and vigorously, you're good to go.

But even if your baking soda isn't potent anymore, you don't need to toss it out. While it may not have enough pep for baking, it's still great for scrubbing and scouring.

Transform your cuisine with these 3 cooking tricks

Baking soda is a vital part of pie crusts and other baked goods. But that's not all this amazing ingredient is good for. These simple kitchen hacks will give you a reason to keep your pantry well stocked with baking soda all the time.

Tone down the acidity. Baking soda has long been used to treat heartburn. That's because it's something called a base, or the chemical opposite of an acid. That means it can neutralize the stomach acid that causes heartburn.

And you can do the same in your food, too. Add a tiny pinch to canned tomato sauces or soups to bring down their harsh, acidic bite.

Soften beans faster. If you don't have time to spend simmering dried beans until they're tender and toothsome, reach for a box of baking soda. It raises the pH of your cooking water, which helps break down beans quicker.

Sprinkle in 1/4 teaspoon of baking soda per pound of dried beans to cut down on cooking time. Adding too much may make your beans taste a bit soapy.

Tenderize tough cuts. Baking soda can keep proteins in meat from bonding and tangling together. The result? A tender, juicy cut that won't get too tough when it cooks.

If you want to try it on chicken or beef before you grill it, simply rub the meat with baking soda and let it rest in the fridge for at least three hours. Rinse off the baking soda before seasoning and cooking.

Plan on stir-frying? Toss 1/4 teaspoon of baking soda onto raw shrimp. Keep the mixture in the fridge for up to an hour for a firm, snappy texture. Rinse before cooking.

A closer look
Emergency substitutions

Run out of milk? Used the last onion? No sign of baking powder? Discover no-fail substitutes you should always keep in your pantry. If you know these simple swaps, you'll never again have to make a last-minute run to the grocery store.

Ingredient	Amount	Substitution
baking powder	1 tsp	1/3 tsp baking soda plus 1/2 tsp cream of tartar
bread crumbs	any	equal amount potato flakes
broth	1 cup	1 cup water plus 1 tbsp soy sauce
brown sugar	1 cup	1 cup granulated sugar plus 1 tbsp molasses
butter, for baking	1 cup	1 cup applesauce
cream of tartar	1 tsp	1 tsp lemon juice
egg	1 whole	3 tbsp canned chickpea liquid
herbs, fresh	1 tbsp	1 teaspoon dried herbs
honey	1 cup	1 1/4 cup sugar plus 1/3 cup water
lard	1 cup	7/8 cup vegetable oil
lemon juice	1 tsp	1/2 tsp vinegar
mayonnaise	any	equal amount mashed avocado
milk	1 cup	1/2 cup evaporated milk plus 1/2 cup water
nutmeg	any	equal amount cinnamon, ginger, or mace
onion, chopped	1/4 cup	1 tsp onion powder
sour cream	any	equal amount plain yogurt
wine	1 cup	1 cup fruit juice plus 1 tbsp vinegar

Chocolate

Your brain on chocolate is sharper than ever

When you think of chocolate, you probably picture a wrapped candy bar. But this food has been around for thousands of years, just not in the form you may have come to expect.

Chocolate is made from the beans of cacao trees, which are native to parts of Central and South America. From its early days in that region to its spread across Europe many years later, people often drank chocolate as a health elixir. And they weren't too far off. Chocolate possesses many health benefits. Read more about how it can assist your brain.

The power of cacao on cognition. Don't just feel younger, be younger, too. Slow your aging by improving your memory and brain function with these foods. It's as simple as choosing dark chocolate or other cacao-dense delights. Researchers have been busy at work studying the effects of dark chocolate on brain function, and the results are promising.

Some research suggests that chocolate rich in cacao could improve verbal memory, mental flexibility, and other cognitive functions. The key here is to pick a dark chocolate that features a high cacao content. Going with a higher percentage, like 85% or more, can dramatically increase the amount of flavonoids you get.

Flavonoids work like antioxidants and may be behind the healthful benefits of dark chocolate, so you want as much as you can get. However, you should still eat chocolate in moderation as it contains a significant amount of fat and carbohydrates.

Munch on this good mood food to fight the blues. Feel yourself drawn to the candy counter when you're down? A treat might actually be just what the doctor ordered. If you choose the right one, that is. Research suggests that dark chocolate is up to the task.

Some studies have shown that people who regularly eat dark chocolate report fewer depressive symptoms. The champion behind the results — flavonoids and other polyphenols. These compounds have anti-inflammatory and antioxidant properties, which may support your brain and mood.

Skim off your stress levels. Chronic stress is a risk factor for big-name conditions like high blood pressure, anxiety, and heart disease. When your body experiences stress, it releases a hormone called cortisol. Lowering your stress hormones levels, including that of cortisol, may influence your body's reactions to stress. Flavonoids might help lower these levels.

To test it out, researchers asked participants to eat dark chocolate with either 500 milligrams of flavonoids or little to no flavonoids. After four weeks, the participants who ate high-flavonoid chocolate had lower cortisol levels than before.

Banish wrinkles with a surprising treat

Wrinkles, whether you love or hate them, are one clear sign of aging. They typically start appearing in your early 40s as your skin loosens and loses its elasticity. Fortunately, scientists have been studying how to slow skin aging.

One study followed a group of women over 40 for six months. Some of the participants drank a beverage with 320 milligrams of cocoa flavanols every day while the other got a drink without cocoa. At the beginning of the study, all of the women had visible wrinkles. Afterward, wrinkles and skin elasticity had improved in the women who drank the cocoa compared to the placebo.

Flavanols are a type of flavonoid found in cocoa and chocolate. These nutrients can help protect your skin from damaging UV radiation. Flavanols are also what scientists theorize are behind cocoa's positive effect on skin aging.

 Boost the benefits

Want to start your day off on the right foot? Believe it or not, eating a little bit of chocolate at breakfast time might be the boost you need.

In a new study, scientists examined the effects of milk chocolate in the morning and nighttime on a small group of participants.

They found that even though the postmenopausal women in the study increased their calories with chocolate, they didn't gain weight. In fact, the results suggest that eating chocolate in the one-hour window after waking up could actually help burn body fat and reduce glucose levels.

"Our findings highlight that not only 'what' but also 'when' we eat can impact physiological mechanisms involved in the regulation of body weight," says Frank Scheer, Ph.D., one of the lead researchers.

The scientists theorize that the chocolate reduced hunger, so although this sweet added calories, the participants didn't eat as many other calories.

This candy crushes cardiovascular disease

Nothing good came of munching on sweets in the Brothers Grimm story "Hansel and Gretel." Fortunately, that fairy tale doesn't hold true in the real world. In fact, having a little chocolate each week could actually improve your life, and not just because it quells your sweet cravings. This treat could bolster your heart and blood vessels.

Chocolate's at the helm of heart healing. A heart-shaped box of chocolates is an iconic gift on Valentine's Day. But you may be surprised to hear that these candies could help your real heart. In the last few years, researchers analyzed the data from 23 studies that examined the effects of eating chocolate on heart health.

This large pool of information revealed that eating chocolate might be associated with a lower risk of heart disease. That's great news as cardiovascular diseases are the No. 1 cause of death across the globe. The researchers pinned the best amount of chocolate to eat a week at about 45 grams. That's about 1.5 ounces or four squares of the average Lindt or Ghirardelli dark chocolate bar.

Wrinkles, heart attacks, stroke, memory loss — chocolate is the magic "pill" that tastes good, too. But how much do you need? The amount used in studies varies since flavonoid content depends on processing. However, one review says you may lose heart benefits if you eat more than 100 grams — or a 3.5-ounce bar — a week.

So where do all these heart-healthy benefits come from? Experts believe that flavanols like epicatechin, catechin, and procyanidin offer heart protection through powerful antioxidant and anti-inflammatory action, among others.

Stave off stroke with a delicious delicacy. Indulge in eating one of these treats every day and you could reduce your risk of stroke and open up your artery walls. In one review, researchers concluded that 50 grams of chocolate in a week is linked to a 14% lower risk of stroke.

The same flavanols that protect against heart disease stymie strokes in a similar manner. They're also antiplatelets, meaning they can help stop blood cells from sticking together and forming a clot.

Despite these benefits of chocolate rich in flavanols, be careful not to overdo it. Eating too much sugary chocolate can still create other health risks, like weight gain.

 Kitchen hacks

Delicious chocolate can become off-putting when its exterior looks white and dusty. Don't worry, it's still perfectly safe to eat. What you're looking at could be a fat bloom, making your chocolate look waxy, or a sugar bloom, which may make your candy feel gritty. They happen when fat or sugar move to the exterior of the chocolate and crystallize.

Dodge these unpleasantries with temperature and moisture control. Keep your chocolate in a cool, dry place away from light. The temperature sweet spot is around 64 degrees. Avoid popping your chocolate into the fridge or freezer if possible. But if you must, cover it in plastic warp first to protect against condensation. Then however you decide to store it, seal it in an airtight container.

This will give your chocolate a longer life. Dark chocolate will stay fresh for about two years. The life span of milk chocolate is shorter at about one year.

Hot cocoa could offer sweet relief for walking pain

Peripheral artery disease (PAD) affects more than 8.5 million people over the age of 40 across the country. Pain, cramps, and weakness in the leg muscles while walking are just some of the most common symptoms. But there are few treatments to improve walking ability for people with this condition. A recent small study of cocoa and PAD could change all that.

When you have PAD, your arteries narrow and reduce blood flow from your heart to your legs. So what can help? Flavanols.

This cocoa compound may improve blood flow and help lower blood pressure.

Best of all, this theory worked when put to the test. The study participants who had a flavanol-rich cocoa drink three times a day for six months were able to walk farther in their six-minute walking test than those who didn't. Those who drank the cocoa beverage also had better calf muscle function and blood flow to their legs. Further research is needed because of the small study size, but these findings could be useful for future treatment options.

Tasty techniques to make dark confections less bitter

Language experts believe the word chocolate comes from the Aztec name for a bitter drink called xocoatl, which they brewed from cacao beans. But never fear, you can mask the bitterness of high-cacao chocolate with these sweet tricks.

- Add salt. You won't actually make chocolate any sweeter with salt, but it can help block out some of the bitterness.

- Sample other sweetness. Pair your dark delicacy with your favorite fruits like strawberries, bananas, or pears. The chocolate's bitterness makes the fruit taste even sweeter.

- Get a little nutty. Kick up flavor and texture interest with nuts.

- Turn up the heat. Ever heard of Mexican hot chocolate? It's spiced up with cinnamon, nutmeg, and even chilies sometimes. The spiciness of these other ingredients give your palate ample distraction.

- Pair with contrasting flavors. Cheese is a perfect match for dark chocolate's bitterness. Aged cheeses like Gouda and havarti, especially, provide perfect balance.

Honey

2 reasons to ditch sugar for this sweeter substitute

The average American devours a whopping 57 pounds of added sugar every year. That's well over 100,000 calories. But if you want to cut back on sugar without going cold turkey, all you have to do is make one change. Some experts say swapping out refined sugar for a smaller amount of honey could be the key to a healthier lifestyle.

Lower your cholesterol and lose weight with a single switch. To test honey versus sugar, researchers divided 60 volunteers into two groups. Half the participants drank a cup of water mixed with about 2 1/2 ounces of honey daily. The others drank a cup of water with 2 1/2 ounces of sucrose — or table sugar — every day.

At the end of six weeks, researchers found that the honey group had lower total and LDL cholesterol. However, the sugar eaters actually had higher cholesterol levels than they did when the study began.

Another small study found that adding honey gradually over eight weeks without changing overall calorie intake lowered cholesterol and weight in people with diabetes.

Want to trade sugar for honey? Remember this advice. Unfortunately, making the switch isn't as straightforward as swapping out a tablespoon of sugar for a tablespoon of honey. That's because honey is much denser than sugar, so each tablespoon actually packs in more calories.

A good rule of thumb is to use about half, or even a third, as much honey by volume as you would for sugar. That means if you normally sweeten your morning coffee with a tablespoon of sugar, start with a single teaspoon of honey.

And if you want to swap out honey for sugar in your cookies, cakes, and other baked goods? Substitute 1/2 cup of honey per cup of sugar. You'll need to dial back the liquids in the recipe by about 1/4 cup, too.

How to guarantee you're getting the real deal

Buying a bottle of honey should be a simple process. But if you head down to the grocery store and grab the first one you see, you might be in for a rude surprise. Some unscrupulous companies cut their honey with corn syrup or other sweeteners to lower their costs. Here are two ways to avoid getting fleeced.

- Make sure it's coming from close to home. You're less likely to go wrong if you buy honey that's made in the USA. And if it's from a local producer, even better.

- Get your honey straight from the source. Beekeeping has become increasingly common, and many bee-keepers sell their goods at local farmers markets. The American Beekeeping Federation also keeps a direc-tory of local beekeeping associations. Go online to *abfnet.org/page/states* and click on your state to find one near you.

Caught a cold? Swap the usual care for an all-natural solution

Searching for relief from a hacking cough, runny nose, and sore throat can seem almost impossible at times. You try just about every over-the-counter med at your local pharmacy, only to find that your symptoms are still hanging on. But the answer may already be hidden away in your kitchen.

A new analysis, published in *BMJ Evidence-Based Medicine*, examined 14 studies that compared honey — including preparations that had honey as an ingredient — to common drugs for soothing upper respiratory tract symptoms. The authors found that honey was better at easing cough severity and frequency as well as overall symptoms.

Want to whip up your own cough-soothing solution? Simply mix 1 to 2 teaspoons of honey into a cup of warm water or your favorite tea. Honey will help with coughs, while the H20 will help you stay hydrated.

Though honey is a relatively safe choice, be aware that each teaspoon has about 6 grams of sugar. So don't overdo it.

Sweeten your smile with an unlikely treat

You may think honey is exactly the kind of thing your dentist wants you to avoid. After all, this sticky, sweet confection seems more like it would cause cavities rather than prevent them. But research suggests that certain types of honey could actually help you fight plaque, rejuvenate your gums, and even soothe mouth sores.

The secret ingredient to support your teeth and gums. In one study, young volunteers swished a raw honey, manuka honey, or traditional chlorhexidine mouthwash twice a day for three weeks. Surprisingly, all three mouthwashes lowered the amount of plaque in people's mouths. And all of them encouraged healthier gums.

The traditional antiseptic kind worked the best, but honey was able to keep pace because it has powerful antimicrobial properties. Experts think it fights off the bacteria that cause plaque, gum disease, and even cavities.

Honey mouthwashes may be hard to find in stores and online, but you can make your own by dissolving up to 5 teaspoons of honey into a cup of warm water. Store the mixture in the fridge.

Canker sores? This natural solution can cool the burn. Painful canker sores inside your cheeks or lips could make eating and drinking a nightmare. Even talking when you have one of these ulcers can set your chops on fire. Unfortunately, scientists aren't sure what causes these lesions to crop up on the soft tissues in your mouth.

The good news is they do know a great, natural way to soothe the pain — honey. In a small study, researchers pitted honey against over-the-counter and prescription treatments for canker sores. They found that honey brought faster pain relief and helped the sores heal quicker.

Want to try it yourself? Volunteers dabbed a small amount of honey directly on the ulcers four times each day.

 Bright idea

Fruit flies buzzing around your kitchen are a huge nuisance. Obviously, you don't want these pesky bugs to infest your fruit and veggies.

At the same time, you surely don't want to spray your whole kitchen with potentially toxic fly killers. So instead of resorting to harsh commercial sprays from the store, try this natural solution.

Fill up a small bowl with a few spoonfuls of honey, a generous helping of vinegar, and a touch of dish soap. Cover it tightly with plastic wrap. Next, use a fork or knife to poke a few holes in the plastic so bugs can crawl through.

They'll be attracted to the sweet, sticky solution of honey and vinegar. But the soap won't allow them to land on the surface of the mixture, so they'll fall in and get trapped.

A closer look
Sugar and other sweeteners

Sugar, sugar, everywhere. Americans eat an average of about 19 teaspoons of added sugar every day. But the American Heart Association (AHA) recommends that men eat no more than 9 teaspoons a day, and women have no more than 6 teaspoons. Quite the difference.

Follow the advice of the AHA and limit or cut out the top source of added sugar — sugar-sweetened beverages. For starters, they can be one of the most dangerous foods for your bowel, having been linked to an increased risk of colorectal cancer. Plus, they don't fill you up the way food does, making you crave more calories. Use these tips to slash how much sugar is in your diet.

Simple sugar swaps. Alternative sweeteners have gotten bad press, but science now finds that they're generally safe. Using artificial sweeteners in moderation could help you avoid the negatives of regular table sugar like diabetes and weight gain. They add very few calories to your diet, and since they're sweeter than sugar, you don't need as much. But beware, they could backfire by triggering your appetite.

- Aspartame. About 200 times sweeter than sugar, aspartame has about the same calorie content per gram, but because it's so sweet you can use less for the same taste. Just don't bake with it since heat causes it to lose sweetness.

- Stevia. This sweetener comes from the leaves of the stevia plant native to South America. A bitter aftertaste is signature to stevia, so it's often blended with an additional sweetener.

  And here's something surprising, but true. Researchers have found that compounds in stevia may help lower blood sugar and blood pressure. So why not switch your sugary soda for one with stevia next time you're at the grocery store.

- Saccharin. This artificial sweetener doesn't have calories but may leave an aftertaste. Saccharin won't lose its sweetness in high heat, so you can use it for cooking and baking. About 2 teaspoons of the Sweet'N Low brand of saccharin will get you the sweetness of 1/4 cup of sugar.

- Sucralose. Unlike other sweeteners, sucralose is made from sugar. Its sweetness has just been chemically enhanced to 600 times that of sugar with almost no calories. That may make its flavor more desirable than other sweeteners.

  Plus, there's no aftertaste. You can use it when baking or cooking. Sucralose in the form of granulated Splenda, for example, subs at a 1-to-1 ratio with sugar.

Size down your sugar intake. You don't have to quit cold turkey. In fact, you can minimize withdrawals and cravings by slowly making swaps. Examine the added sugars in what you eat regularly. Then find tasty substitutes for sugary fare.

Herbal tea or seltzer may hit the spot in place of a sweetened soda. Add flavor to your dishes using extracts, like almond or vanilla, or switch up the palate with spices like ginger or cinnamon. Applesauce is an excellent substitute in baking, and you can use 1 cup of it in place of 1 cup of sugar.

Recognize hidden sweeteners. In order to cut added sugar from your diet, you need to be able to identify it. Even foods that claim to be sugar-free might have an artificial sweetener.

When reading food labels look for ingredients with the word "sugar," "nectar," or "syrup." Also check for words ending in "-ose," like sucrose and dextrose.

Other added sugars include honey, molasses, sweet sorghum, and cane juice. It's important to remember that "natural" doesn't necessarily mean "good for you."

Nutritional yeast

Bring on the B12 to boost your brainpower

You may think of nutritional yeast as little more than a cheese substitute for health-food freaks. After all, these yellow flakes are called "hippie dust" due to their popularity among people who don't eat meat. But this seasoning is becoming more and more popular, and for a good reason. If you're not stocking your pantry with nutritional yeast, you're missing out on a great source of B vitamins.

Feeling forgetful lately? You might be missing this common nutrient. You may be quick to blame old age if you can't remember where you put your reading glasses or car keys, but a simple vitamin B12 deficiency may be the culprit.

Even if you're already eating plenty of vitamin B12-rich foods — like dairy and meat — you may need to seek out a new source. As you age, your stomach produces less acid, making it harder for your body to break down and absorb the B12 that occurs naturally in food.

> Nutritional yeast is yummy dusted on roasted veggies, stirred into rice, or sprinkled on popcorn. Store it in a cool, dry pantry or the fridge for up to two years.

That's where nutritional yeast comes in. It's often fortified with vitamins that are ready for your body to use straight away, so you can easily absorb plenty of memory-saving B12. And a single serving of fortified nutritional yeast could offer nearly 10 times your daily needs.

A sprinkle of yellow to help beat the blues. Vitamin B12 plays an important role in producing the chemicals your brain needs to regulate your mood. Run low and you run the risk of depression.

A recent study published in *BMC Psychiatry* compared the diets of people with depression to the diets of similar, but otherwise healthy, people. The researchers found that those who had unhealthy eating patterns with foods lower in B12 were more likely to suffer from depression.

Shop smarter — how to pick the perfect flakes

Think all nutritional yeast brands are the same? You couldn't be more wrong. This flavorful seasoning — which is made by cultivating *Saccharomyces cerevisiae* yeast — is sold a few different ways. And depending on which one you buy, you may get wildly different amounts of nutrients.

- If you want to get plenty of nourishment, look for a product that's been fortified with vitamin B12, folic acid, and other nutrients you may be lacking, like iron. Otherwise you'll only get the trace minerals and vitamins that the yeast produces as it grows.

- Protein content varies from brand to brand, so check the label and pay close attention to the serving size. Some brands list a serving as 1/4 cup, while others may say a serving is a tablespoon.

2 ways this savory seasoning helps you stay fit as a fiddle

Investing in your health is of utmost importance if you want to stay active and vigorous well into your senior years. Otherwise, you roll the dice on developing sarcopenia, a disease characterized by weakening muscles, which increases your chances of falls and fractures.

One of the best ways to keep your body buff? Nutritional yeast. This kitchen must-have is packed with two nutrients vital to your fight against sarcopenia.

Be sure you get enough of this important vitamin to stay spry. In a small study, researchers recruited adults who were at least 65 years old and suffered from sarcopenia. Then they matched them with a healthy adult and compared their diets. They discovered that seniors with sarcopenia ate fewer foods rich in B12.

The exact reason behind this vitamin's powers is still unclear, but fortunately experts know how to keep you from running low. A single tablespoon of fortified nutritional yeast could have 4.4 micrograms (mcg) of vitamin B12, well over the recommended 2.4 mcg you need every day.

Want to keep your muscles strong? Pack on the protein. This essential nutrient is the building block for every single cell in your body. You need to get plenty of it if you don't want your muscles to start to fade away and weaken with age.

Experts say you should try to eat at least 20 to 30 grams of protein with each meal. But chowing down on enough protein-rich foods — like meat, beans, and lentils — can be tough as you get older and your appetite wanes. The good news? Adding a little bit of nutritional yeast is a low-cal way to amp up your protein intake. One tablespoon may contain 2 grams of protein while only clocking in at 15 calories.

Guard against disease with a little help from this pantry powerhouse

You may pile your plate high with grains and lentils when you're trying to get your fiber fix. But nutritional yeast is a great — and tasty — way to get a little bit of extra fiber in your meals. And even better, it's loaded with a special type of fiber called beta glucan.

Keep your heart healthy. Studies on the most popular sources of beta glucan, oats and barley, have found that eating beta glucan each day helps lower LDL cholesterol — that's the bad kind. The reason? Experts think this nutrient may block your stomach and intestines from absorbing cholesterol from food.

Boost your immune system. Research has shown that people who took beta glucan — equal to the amount found in about a tablespoon of nutritional yeast — every day were 25% less likely to catch the common cold than people who took a placebo.

This powder doesn't work by fending off harmful germs directly. Instead, scientists think beta glucans help activate your body's natural defenses against disease.

 Watch out

Once you've discovered nutritional yeast, it can be hard to resist the urge to sprinkle this powder on everything. But if you're too gung-ho, you may be met with some unpleasant — or even dangerous — side effects.

- Nutritional yeast is a great source of fiber, but piling it on too quickly may cause digestive issues like bloating and discomfort. Try to add it slowly to your diet if you don't already eat a lot of high-fiber foods.

- These flakes are also high in a compound called tyramine, which is a common trigger for migraines. If you suffer from these debilitating headaches, be careful with nutritional yeast.

- Certain compounds found in this seasoning powder may interfere with prescriptions commonly used to treat diabetes, depression, and pain. Check with your doctor to make sure nutritional yeast won't cause dangerous interactions with any drug you take.

Olive oil

Loosen your brain cogs with this healthy headliner

Feel like the gears in your mind are slowing down or getting stuck? Grease them up with olive oil. Research suggests that this ingredient could guard your memory.

The most common form of dementia among seniors is Alzheimer's disease (AD). AD can impact language, mood, motivation levels, and the ability to take care of yourself. This disorder affects about 5% of people age 65, and its prevalence increases to more than 40% by age 85.

There isn't a cure, so the best you can do is hold off cognitive decline. That's where extra-virgin olive oil (EVOO) comes in. This food is rich in nutrients that support your mind, like fatty acids and antioxidants. EVOO has been connected to lower oxidative stress which may play a role in protecting your brain function.

Dine along the Italian coastline. The delicious Mediterranean diet features lots of fruits, vegetables, fish, and of course, olive oil. Studies have revealed that seniors who follow a Mediterranean diet with extra doses of EVOO show better cognitive function than those on a regular Mediterranean diet. That sure is an encouragement for switching out your vegetable oils with this healthy and tasty choice.

Set your MIND on power-packed plates. Another eating pattern you may be familiar with is the MIND diet. It is a blend of the Mediterranean diet and DASH diet, and it's specifically geared toward protecting, you guessed it, your mind.

One study found that closely following the Mediterranean or DASH diet was associated with fewer cases of AD. The MIND diet, on the other hand, showed protection even when it wasn't adhered to as strictly. The rate of AD for a middle-of-the-road level of following this diet was reduced by about 35%. This remarkable difference was from the food, no drug involved.

And it gets even better. The scientists estimated that those who stuck to the diet the most were a whopping 53% less likely to get AD compared to those who were the least devoted.

The researchers suggest that even making a small change to your diet could dramatically improve your protection against dementia. So eat more MIND diet essentials like leafy greens, berries, whole grains, nuts, beans, and olive oil.

Cancer meets a bitter end via key compounds

Early cancer diagnosis and treatment can improve someone's outcome, but they often still experience side effects. That's why researchers have been looking into plant alternatives that could aid in cancer treatment.

They've discovered compounds that make cancer cells self-destruct. And you may have some in your kitchen right now. These nutrients are found in olive oil, that old reliable ingredient.

Specifically, you want extra-virgin olive oil (EVOO). Other oils that are refined have been stripped of naturally occurring vitamins, polyphenols, and phytosterols. Extra-virgin olive oil, on the other hand, has the highest level of polyphenols. That's important because those micronutrients may be the key to cancer protection.

Polyphenols have strong antioxidant and anti-inflammatory powers that make them cancer fighters. One in particular, called oleuropein, does much of the heavy lifting. Not only does this compound give unprocessed olives their distinct bitter taste, it also has been shown time and again in lab studies to slow the spread of cancer cells and even cause cancer cell death, called apoptosis.

The benefits of compounds in olive oil like oleuropein and oleocanthal aren't limited to one type of cancer, either. Eating higher amounts of EVOO is linked to a lower risk of having any type of cancer, particularly digestive system and breast cancers.

Grocery guru: How to pinpoint the perfect bottle

Bottles upon bottles of olive oil fill grocery store shelves. Here's the right way to choose among them.

- Always pick extra-virgin olive oil. It's higher quality than other olive oils and isn't treated with damaging heat.

- Exposure to light degrades olive oil. Select a bottle made of dark glass or metal.

- Beware of unusually cheap bottles that claim to be products of Italy. They may have actually just gotten packaged there. Instead look for the initials of the country where the olives were grown and pressed. One from a single country is often better quality.

- The fresher you can get, the better, so always check the "best by" date. A "pressed on" or "harvest date" likely indicates a higher quality product.

- The flavor of olive oil can signal how beneficial it is to your health. Oils that are more bitter with a pungent, peppery taste often have higher polyphenol levels.

The heartening powers of liquid gold

Animal fat is a clear loser when it comes to your health. Getting more vegetable fat, however, is associated with a lower risk of stroke. So if you're worried about your heart and blood vessel health, take extra care when choosing cooking oils and condiments. Spoiler alert — extra-virgin olive oil may be the cream of the crop.

Drop your chances of heart havoc with simple switches. Researchers have tied better heart health to eating higher amounts of olive oil, and small swaps might do the trick. The study followed nearly 93,000 men and women over the course of two decades and gathered information about their diet and lifestyle.

> Olive oil is essential for cooking, but it has other household uses, too. You can restore your wooden cutting boards and utensils by rubbing a few drops on them. Or take to your dull furniture with a homemade polish. Mix 2 parts olive oil with 1 part lemon juice, then rub on and wipe dry.

- Trading 1 teaspoon of butter, margarine, mayonnaise, or dairy fat for the same amount of olive oil each day was linked to a 5% lower risk of cardiovascular disease, a group of heart and blood vessel disorders.

- This simple change was also associated with a 7% lower risk of coronary heart disease, which is caused by clogged arteries.

Get extra blood pressure perks with extra-virgin. The long-term force of high blood pressure on your artery walls spells bad news for your health. Olive oil to the rescue.

In a recent study, participants ate either 4 tablespoons of a high-polyphenol extra-virgin olive oil or a low-polyphenol commercial olive oil each day for three weeks. After a two-week washout period, they switched olive oils and repeated the experiment.

The researchers found that the olive oil high in polyphenols decreased systolic blood pressure.

The benefits of extra-virgin olive oil may be due to the antioxidant activity of its polyphenols. So go on. Swirl this liquid gold into creamy soups or homemade dips like hummus.

Fight fractures and flab the tasty way

Pop quiz. Is olive oil made from unripe green olives or ripe black olives? Usually, it's both. This winning combination is a triumph for your taste buds. And there's more. The fusion may also be double trouble for this duo of health concerns.

Rebuild your bone structure. Bone-forming cells called osteoblasts are in charge of building up your skeleton and keeping it strong. Osteoporosis happens when you have an imbalance between bone formation and resorption, the breakdown of your skeleton that leads to lower bone mass and density. This breakdown is controlled by cells called osteoclasts.

Remember it this way: -blasts are bone builders, and -clasts cause cracks. So how do you get more of the builders and less of the other cells? According to lab studies, extra-virgin olive oil (EVOO) might help.

- The polyphenols in EVOO, like oleuropein, caffeic acid, and apigenin, may encourage the creation and activity of osteoblasts. That can lead to bone formation, preservation, and repair.

- These compounds may also block the production of osteoclasts and so decrease bone loss.

Researchers speculate that EVOO compounds may one day prove to be protective against bone conditions like osteoporosis.

Cover all your bases, and slip this oil in with foods that contain bone-boosting calcium and vitamin D. Use it to bake salmon, for instance, or as a base for dressing on your kale salad.

Fight fat with fat. Whittle your waist by eating more fat? It may sound counterintuitive, but a study found that eating the right fatty food might make the difference. Women with excess body fat received daily high-fat breakfasts containing just under 2 tablespoons of soybean oil or EVOO for nine weeks. Those who ate the EVOO lost more fat.

The researchers say a type of monounsaturated fatty acid in EVOO called oleic acid may influence an enzyme that plays a role in weight loss. Authors of other studies supporting olive oil for weight management theorize that it helps people feel fuller.

 Bright idea

And the award for most versatile item in your pantry goes to ... olive oil! Steal it from your cuisine routine, and use it for personal care. You may want to buy a bottle of olive oil specially for your bathroom after you hear these tips.

Olive oil is an excellent moisturizer you can use on your skin. Remedy your cracked heels by exfoliating them with a pumice stone and applying some olive oil. Finish it off by covering your feet with socks and letting them absorb the oil overnight.

You can also use this oil on your hair. It may help prevent breakage and split ends through the power of oleic acid and squalane, two emollients that soften and hydrate. Just make sure to use unrefined, cold-pressed extra-virgin olive oil.

It also works great in place of shaving cream for a smooth finish. You can even coat your razor blades with olive oil to prevent rusting.

A visionary remedy for your eyesight

Is the juice worth the squeeze? Well, yes, if the juice in question comes from squeezing fresh olives. Your eyes will agree that olive juice, aka olive oil, is worth all the effort it takes to get it to your plate.

To understand why, you need to know that inflammation and oxidative stress are two key factors that contribute to AMD, or age-related macular degeneration, an eye disease that affects central vision. And the polyphenols in olive oil may be able to combat both.

- Some of the significant anti-inflammatory effects of olive oil may be influenced by the polyphenol oleocanthal, which behaves similarly to ibuprofen. Just how powerful is it? Experts estimate that about 4 tablespoons of olive oil has enough oleocanthal to provide about 10% of the pain relief of the ibuprofen in your cabinet.

- Olive oil polyphenols like hydroxytyrosol also have antioxidant activity. Some research has shown that they can protect against oxidative damage in eye cells.

Interestingly, the main effect olive oil seems to have on macular degeneration is reserved for late-stage AMD. At this point in the condition, you may have a blurry spot in the center of your vision that could increase in size. Straight lines may start looking wavy or crooked, and colors can appear less bright than before. You might also have more difficulty seeing in low light.

Your diet may be one way to lower your risk of this severe form of AMD. And that's where olive oil comes into play. It is a major facet of the Mediterranean diet and often gets some of the credit for the eating plan's health benefits. The Mediterranean diet has been linked to a lower occurrence of many conditions, including AMD.

More than that, a study with over 600 participants found that eating olive oil regularly was associated with decreased rates of late AMD. The exact amount of olive oil was not measured, so more research is still needed, but scientists think these results could be promising.

Fibromyalgia plan add-on to tame the pain

Doctors still don't know a whole lot about fibromyalgia. This chronic, often disabling condition is characterized by pain spread widely throughout the body. That includes joint stiffness, burning skin, headaches, and more. The origins are unclear, but scientists hypothesize that an increase in oxidative stress and inflammation are likely involved.

A variety of medication has been used to treat fibromyalgia, but none have been completely effective on their own. For that reason, doctors and patients are turning to a combined approach of drug and natural treatment. This includes diet changes, and it's why extra-virgin olive oil may be useful in managing this condition.

Olive oil offers protection from inflammation. In particular, one of its components, hydroxytyrosol, may play a significant role. A recent study dove into the cellular makeup of people with fibromyalgia to get a closer look. Scientists treated their cells in a lab with hydroxytyrosol. They found that this compound had a beneficial impact, including protein changes related to oxidative stress and inflammation.

As such, the researchers believe that a diet high in hydroxytyrosol could be a helpful method of managing fibromyalgia. Don't get ahead of yourself, though. This isn't a cure-all, and more research is needed, especially since hydroxytyrosol is just a small part of olive oil.

Vinegar

Ordinary food with fat-fighting powers protects your heart

Heart disease costs Americans an estimated $363 billion every year. To put that into perspective, if you saved $10,000 every day it would take almost 100,000 years to stock away that much cash. Hold on to your purse strings by doing what you can to guard your heart and keep it healthy. That's where vinegar comes in.

A dash of vinegar may help trim your waistline. Your heart has to pump blood all throughout your body. The harder it has to work, the bigger your risk of developing heart disease. If you're overweight or obese, your heart may be pumping overtime to get the job done.

The silver lining — a small study found that vinegar may help people lose weight and prevent fat from accumulating in their bodies. Japanese researchers recruited obese adults and asked them to either drink a little bit of vinegar or a placebo every day. After 12 weeks, they discovered that the vinegar-drinkers lost more weight and body fat than the people who took the placebo.

They believe acetic acid may be partly responsible for the results. This acid, which gives vinegar its characteristic taste, may encourage your body to suppress fat formation.

It's easy to add vinegar to your diet at home, too. Volunteers who lost the most weight drank about 2 tablespoons of apple cider vinegar every day. They mixed about a tablespoon with water and drank it after breakfast, and did the same after dinner.

Curb cholesterol with this uncommon combination. Think of high cholesterol a bit like traffic jams in your arteries. These fatty deposits build up in your blood vessels over time, creating blockages where only a few blood cells can squeeze through at a time. Not only does your heart have to work harder to make up for the slower flow of blood, but these cholesterol deposits can break off and cause heart attacks, too. Early evidence suggests vinegar could help keep cholesterol levels from getting out of control.

In a small trial, scientists recruited 50 adults with high cholesterol and randomly assigned them to drink a placebo or a cocktail made up of date vinegar and garlic juice. At the end of the seven-week study, researchers discovered that only those who drank the vinegar beverage had drops in cholesterol levels.

Again, researchers think acetic acid deserves some of the credit. That's encouraging since, though date vinegar may be hard to come by, all vinegars contain acetic acid.

 Watch out

Vinegar is a relatively safe food, but it's not for everyone. These two common conditions may mean you need to steer clear of vinegar.

- Chronic kidney disease. Your kidneys work hard to filter out extra acid from your body. But if they're not working at 100%, you don't want to strain them by adding loads of acidic foods and drinks — like vinegar — to your daily diet. Some research suggests that people with chronic kidney disease have an increased risk of kidney failure when they follow a diet loaded with acidic foods.

- Heartburn. Acidic foods are a common trigger for acid reflux. It's best to introduce vinegar slowly if you think it may cause heartburn or other digestive woes.

Use this common ingredient to beat the blood sugar blues

Before modern diabetes medicine hit the market, people used to guzzle vinegar to help keep their blood sugar under control. Now, research suggests that this time-honored folk remedy may have some solid science behind it.

Blunt blood sugar spikes when you eat. Keeping blood sugar levels steady is a constant struggle for people with diabetes. If glucose levels rise too high it can cause fatigue, headaches, and blurred vision. In rare cases, high blood sugar levels increase the risk of a potentially fatal condition called diabetic ketoacidosis, which causes blood to become dangerously acidic.

Research suggests that sipping on vinegar could help prevent sugar spikes. Greek researchers asked volunteers with diabetes to drink 2 tablespoons of vinegar mixed with just over a tablespoon of water or a placebo five minutes before a meal. The study revealed that vinegar kept blood sugar levels from skyrocketing after eating. Experts think it may help your body use insulin more effectively to process sugars.

Keep fasting glucose levels down. A recent review suggests that vinegar could help lower fasting blood glucose levels of people with diabetes. That's great news since long-term high blood sugar levels are linked with heart, kidney, and nerve damage.

In another study, healthy participants who were at risk for type 2 diabetes saw the same benefits after drinking a tablespoon of apple cider vinegar mixed into a cup of water at mealtime twice daily. Completely doable.

Before you start gulping down vinegar every day, though, talk to your doctor. Too much vinegar can cause certain prescription drugs, including diabetes medication, to be less effective.

Watch out

Some people swear by apple cider vinegar as a cure-all for just about any health concern. Many even claim it's a sour solution for gas, bloating, and other tummy troubles. However, no evidence supports vinegar for treating an upset stomach. In fact, experts warn that this drink may cause more harm than good.

Research suggests that sipping on cider vinegar actually slows down the rate at which food passes through your intestines. That's bad news if you're prone to bloating and other digestive problems. It gives the food more time to stay in your gut, which increases the amount of gas produced.

Savvy shopping tips that could save you a bundle

One of the most expensive vinegars in the world — aged balsamic from Modena, Italy — can sell for well over $300 a bottle. It takes hundreds of pounds of grapes and 25 to 50 years just to make a small amount of this exotic vinegar, hence the price tag.

While you may not want to spend hundreds of dollars to get a bottle of pricey balsamic, you may desire something a bit nicer than the plain vinegar you use to wipe down your bathtub. Here's a simple shopping guide to help you pick something delicious that won't break the bank.

Scan the ingredient list to get the real deal. Looking for a vinegar to use in a salad dressing? Opt for a bottle packed with first-class flavor.

Some companies sell higher-priced products that aren't much more than cheap, white distilled vinegar cut with added colors and flavorings. To get a higher quality bottle, look for brands that have nothing more than the base ingredient and water in the product label.

Decide if you're going to go with filtered or not. You may see some cider vinegars advertised as unfiltered. These often have a slightly punchier flavor, but they may not be a wise choice if you don't use a lot of vinegar.

The filtration process removes the live microorganisms that ferment alcohol into acetic acid. Leave them in the bottle and the fermentation process can continue in your pantry, which may cause vinegars to develop unpleasant, yeasty flavors.

To banish the funky smell of vinegar, do this

Not everyone is a fan of vinegar's rather pungent odor. If you can't stand the smell, use these simple tips to reap all the benefits of its cleaning powers without suffering through the stench.

- Making a cleaning solution? Mix it with some better-smelling stuff. Steeping dried herbs with white vinegar can impart pleasant scents. Stir a few pinches of your favorite herbs into a cup of vinegar and let it sit for several hours or days before you use it. You can add a few drops of lemon juice to it for an even fresher smell.

- Neutralize the vinegar with a bit of baking soda. If you use vinegar to sop up a stain on your rug, for example, sprinkle baking soda over it afterward to help keep your carpet from smelling sour. Let it sit for at least 15 minutes before vacuuming.

3 home hacks to help you make the most of your vinegar

A vinegar and baking soda blend to clear clogged drains may be one of the trendiest ways to put vinegar to use. But that's not all this pantry superstar is good for. Here are a few more ways you can solve household problems without spending a fortune on new supplies.

Make a natural ant repellent. Noticed a line of ants streaming into your kitchen? You don't need to resort to toxic sprays to keep these invaders from raiding your pantry. Instead, simply concoct a spray of equal parts vinegar and water. Spritz it on the ants and any areas where you see them coming into the house. Do it three times a week.

The smell of vinegar will block the pheromones these insects use to find their way into your home. If the ant problem is particularly bad, don't dilute the solution.

Kill weeds in your garden without harsh sprays. Keeping your lawn and garden weed-free can be tough work, especially if you don't want to use dangerous pesticides. A simple solution of vinegar and dish soap can tackle tough weeds.

Just mix half a gallon of vinegar with half a cup of salt and a teaspoon of dish soap. Spray it onto the leaves of any weeds in your garden, taking care to avoid getting it on your grass or plants. In no time, you'll have weed-free walkways and more.

Refresh your rusty old tools with a vinegar soak. If your wrenches or screwdrivers are covered in rust, you don't need to toss them out. You may be able to revive them by soaking them in a tub of vinegar and salt.

Use 1/4 cup of salt per 4 cups of vinegar. Let the tools sit for one to three days until the surface rust has loosened, then scrub them clean and dry them thoroughly before storing.

Ingenious cooking tricks you've never tried

Want to use your vinegars for more than just tidying up around the kitchen? Adding a splash of this common pantry ingredient to your next dish could make it the star of your church potluck. Here are four ways to transform your cooking with a simple bottle of vinegar.

Keep your pie crust flaky. A touch of white vinegar in your pie dough can — in theory — inhibit gluten development, which gives you a tender, crispier crust. Even more importantly, vinegar may make it more difficult to overwork pie dough and turn it into a gluey mess. The extra acid also helps stop dough from turning gray and oxidizing if you need to leave it in the fridge for a few hours.

Prevent green beans from turning to mush. If you boil or simmer green beans for too long, they'll become soft and fall apart. That's because high heat causes pectin — which gives structure to the cells of vegetables — to break down into mush. But adjusting the acidity of your cooking liquid with a few spoonfuls of your favorite vinegar can slow down the chemical process. Your green beans will turn slightly brown, but they'll stay snappy and crisp even after they've been stewing for a while.

Stop your pasta from sticking together. Forget about adding oil to your pasta water to keep it from clumping together. Oil isn't as dense as water, so it simply floats on top of the cooking water and does little to prevent noodles from sticking to each other. To keep your pasta from turning into a starchy lump, pour in a tablespoon of vinegar. Increasing the amount of acid in your pasta water prevents noodles from releasing as much starch, so they won't stick together.

Poach or boil your eggs to perfection. Ever drop an egg into a pot of boiling water only to see wisps of egg white leaching out into the pot? Not only will you have an unpleasant mess to clean up later, but your boiled eggs will have a massive chunk missing when you crack them open.

Add a dash of vinegar to the cooking water to stop eggs from escaping through tiny cracks in their shells. And if you're poaching them, it will help the eggs hold their shape while they simmer.

Soothe aching, creaking joints with this folk remedy

You already know that one 99-cent bottle of vinegar can help you unclog your drain, control your blood sugar, repel pesky ants, and make a flaky pie crust. But did you know that many people swear by this home remedy to help them ease their arthritis pain?

Some people claim that apple cider vinegar contains anti-inflammatory properties to help soothe the pain from arthritis. You won't find any scientific evidence supporting these benefits, but you can try it for yourself to see if it helps relieve your sore joints.

Drink 2 teaspoons of cider vinegar mixed into a glass of water each day. Or soak in a bath of warm water and 1 to 2 cups of vinegar.

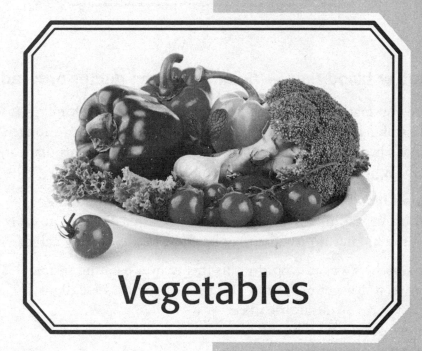

Vegetables

Beets

Better blood flow — 'juice' what the doctor ordered

Are you marching to the "beet" of your own drum? Drinking a glass of delicious beet juice might make that strut much stronger. That's because beets are chock-full of natural chemicals that can improve your blood flow and brain health.

Keep blood pressure woes at bay. Could the fountain of youth be waiting for you in a glass of beet juice? Quite possibly — the nitrates it provides may hold the key to healthy aging.

Researchers set out to prove this theory by separating people between the ages of 70 and 80 into two groups. One drank 2.5 ounces of nitrate-rich beet juice twice a day. The other group drank the same amount of juice with the nitrates taken out.

After 10 days, the scientists tested the saliva samples of all the seniors. They found that the participants who drank the nitrate-rich juice had higher levels of "good" bacteria that promote healthy blood vessels and improve cognition. Not only that, those seniors saw their systolic blood pressure drop by an average of 5 points.

> Here's a trick to peeling beets. Cook them first — boiling and roasting are common methods — so that the skins slide right off after cooling. You can avoid ending up with pink-stained hands by donning a pair of gloves or use a paper towel to remove the outer layer.

"We are really excited about our findings, which have important implications for healthy aging," says Professor Anni Vanhatalo, a researcher at the College of Life and Environmental Sciences at the University of Exeter. "Maintaining the healthy oral micro-biome in the long term might slow down the negative vascular and cognitive changes associated with aging."

Boost your brainpower. You'll want to load up on a tall glass of beet juice if you're looking to protect your brain from the ravages of dementia.

In a two-day study, seniors ate either low-nitrate foods or high-nitrate foods that included nearly 17 ounces of beet juice with breakfast. Researchers then took an MRI of their brains.

The test revealed that the people who drank the beet juice had increased blood flow to areas of the brain linked to dementia and other cognitive issues. Why is that important? Your blood supplies your brain with the glucose and oxygen it needs to function properly.

So march on, and enjoy some delicious beet juice for better brain health.

Beauty and the beet: 6 surprising health benefits of greens

Think twice before tossing those hearty leaves that sprout from fresh bundles of beets. These yummy greens may not get as much attention as other leafy vegetables, but they certainly deserve their time in the limelight. After all, beet greens are loaded with the following nutrients that provide a host of health benefits.

- Vitamin A is essential for eye health and lowers the risk of age-related eye diseases.

- Vitamin C plays an important role in healthy immunity and has anti-aging effects on your skin.

- Vitamin K works with vitamin D to help your body absorb calcium and maintain strong bones.

- Potassium maintains healthy bones and helps keep blood pressure under control.

- Magnesium keeps the immune system strong and supports heart health.

- Manganese may increase both bone mineral density and the formation of new bone.

Just like their vibrant red roots, beet greens are versatile and can be prepared in a variety of delicious ways. You can saute them in olive oil and garlic for a tasty side dish. Or add them to your favorite cubed vegetables and herbs when making a hearty soup or stew. You can also sprinkle apple slices and feta cheese over beet greens if you're in the mood for a tasty salad.

Blending beet roots into a smoothie or juice? Throw the greens into the puree for an extra boost of nutrition.

Just make sure you wash beet greens thoroughly before eating. You can store them in a resealable plastic bag in the fridge for up to four days before using.

Kitchen hacks

Juicing beets at home allows you to easily enjoy their nutritional goodness. If you don't have a juicer, a blender can do the trick.

Start by washing and peeling two to three medium-sized fresh beets. Then chop them finely and put them in your blender with 1/4 cup of water. Blend on high. If the texture is too thick, add small amounts of water. You can add apple, carrots, berries, or bananas for extra flavor and nutrition.

Use a fine-mesh strainer or cheesecloth to remove the pulp if you prefer a thinner consistency. But remember, keeping the pulp will boost the drink's fiber content. Any leftover beet juice can be safely stored in an airtight container in the refrigerator for two days.

Broccoli

Don't miss these 3 astonishing health benefits

Thomas Jefferson was more than a Founding Father. He was also a self-taught architect and avid gardener who liked to experiment with Italian-imported broccoli seeds. Jefferson's keen interest in growing broccoli could make him one of the first Americans to study this amazing veggie. Here's why you should be eating more of it.

Broccoli gets to the heart of the issue. Looking for ways to keep your ticker in tiptop shape? Consider all that broccoli can do.

- Lowers your cholesterol. Most people don't get enough fiber, which is only found in plant foods. One simple way to fix that is to add more broccoli to your diet. It's a great source of fiber, which helps lower cholesterol levels. This, in turn, keeps your heart pumping better.

- Heads off blood vessel damage in people with diabetes. Researchers tested the effects of sulforaphane — an antioxidant in broccoli — on blood vessel cells damaged by high glucose levels. They found that the sulfur-rich compound helped protect the blood vessels by fighting off rogue molecules that would have caused further harm.

- Keeps your arteries flowing freely. Did you know that calcium deposits can build up in your blood vessels? This can significantly increase your risk of heart disease. But broccoli may keep this from happening. A study of more than 680 senior women found that those who ate at least 1.6 ounces of cruciferous vegetables daily — say, 1/2 cup of raw broccoli — were less likely to have extensive amounts of calcium in the blood vessel leading away from the heart than those who ate little to none each day.

Boost your immune system. Your immune system is turbo-charged when you fuel it with great nutrition. Choosing to eat foods like broccoli is a simple strategy for helping you stay strong when fighting off illness and keeping harmful germs at bay.

Why? Broccoli is a rich source of vitamin C, which helps support your immune system. A cup of raw, chopped broccoli will give you 135% of the daily recommended amount of this important nutrient. Wow!

But there's more. Scientists think that the sulforaphane in broccoli can inhibit the growth of the harmful *Helicobacter pylori* bacteria that can cause gastritis and peptic ulcers.

Broccoli is a descendent of the magnificent wild mustard plant, which is also the proud parent of cauliflower, kohlrabi, Brussels sprouts, kale, and cabbage. How can this be? It was all done through selective breeding. Broccoli, for example, was developed from the wild mustard plant's stems and flower buds.

Help prevent cancer with these compounds. Studies have found that a high intake of cruciferous vegetables — think broccoli, cauliflower, and bok choy — is linked to a lower risk of cancer. How is that? Some evidence suggests that broccoli's cancer-fighting properties are attributed to compounds called glucosinolates that break down into anti-inflammatory powerhouses.

Other research based on animal and lab studies suggests that the sulforaphane in broccoli can prevent breast cancer cells from forming and multiplying. Moreover, when this compound is applied topically, it may also protect skin from the harmful UV rays that can cause cancer.

Boost the benefits

Want to get the most nutrition from broccoli? Then don't microwave or boil it. Doing so leeches out the vitamin C in this tasty veggie. Instead, gently steam broccoli for two or three minutes to retain as much vitamin C as possible.

Here's another trick to boosting broccoli's nutritional power. Finely chop this veggie up and let it sit for 30 to 90 minutes. This activates an enzyme in the broccoli that increases the amount of sulforaphane that you get. Steam for easy chewing or eat raw with your favorite hummus for a crunchy snack.

Super sulforaphane eases achy joints

Having osteoarthritis — a degeneration of the joint cartilage and underlying bone — can take a significant toll on your life. Joint pain, stiffness, and swelling in your hands, feet, hips, and knees can make it hard to get around as well as you used to.

But what if someone told you that eating just one green veggie could slow or even prevent the progression of this disease? Yup — broccoli to the rescue. It's rich in a nutrient called sulforaphane that blocks the enzymes — the proteins that speed up chemical reactions in your body — that cause joints to deteriorate.

Researchers from the University of East Anglia in the United Kingdom tested these findings on 40 people with osteoarthritis who were due to have total knee replacement surgery. Over two weeks, half of them ate 3 1/2 ounces each day of a specially engineered broccoli that was extra high in compounds that get broken down into sulforaphane. The rest didn't.

At the end of the study, the scientists found that the broccoli-eating group saw an increase in protein levels in their joint fluid.

They say the study demonstrates that joints can soak up molecules from broccoli that protect them from osteoarthritis damage.

So eat your broccoli. It may be a simple way to help you dance through life.

 Bright idea

You can choose among multiple types of broccoli. Calabrese is the type you may know best. It's the green broccoli with thick stalks and tightly packed florets. Calabrese is the most common variety of this vegetable in the United States.

Broccolini, a cross between broccoli and Chinese kale, has a more delicate design with thin stalks, small florets, and a few leaves. It's milder, and has a sweeter taste, than Calabrese broccoli.

Arcadia broccoli is cold resistant, so you might be more likely to spot this one in the winter with its smaller, purplish-green crowns. You'll love it if you're a fan of raw veggies — Arcadia broccoli has a wonderful crunch.

Lastly, purple cauliflower is technically a type of broccoli. Supermarkets often sell it alongside white cauliflower but you'll recognize it by its bright purple florets.

---

6 nutrients move these 'mini trees' to the top of your grocery list

"When it's dinnertime, I got somethin' you should try," sings the rock-rap band Rocket Surgeons on a secret track. "It's crunchy, green, and yummy, and it's 'bout to blow your mind." What are they jamming about? Broccoli, of course.

It's low in calories, delicious, and packed with disease-fighting nutrients. Here are six reasons why, just like the Rocket Surgeons, you too will be "excited and delighted at the sight of mini trees."

- Broccoli is high in fiber, a vital nutrient that's missing from most people's plates way too often. Fiber offers protective benefits related to digestion, weight, diabetes, stroke, high blood pressure, and heart disease.

- It's an excellent source of vitamin K, which is crucial for healthy blood clotting and works alongside vitamin D to keep your bones and teeth strong. In fact, 1 cup of chopped raw broccoli contains about 93 micrograms of vitamin K. That's more than 100% of the amount women need daily and 77% of what men require.

- That same cup of broccoli contains 14% of the folate you need each day. This B vitamin is necessary for making DNA and dividing cells. And research shows that getting enough in your diet may lower the risk of depression and several forms of cancer.

- Broccoli is also a source of powerful antioxidants, compounds that help fend off free radicals that can damage your cells and lead to disease. One of these is called sulforaphane, which is found in all cruciferous vegetables but is especially active in broccoli. It may help lower high cholesterol and blood sugar levels, as well as defend against cancer.

- It also contains lutein and zeaxanthin, two powerful antioxidants that are especially good for vision. These compounds are actually found in your eyes, where they protect them from damaging blue light and help your sight — so eat up.

- Finally, broccoli has an antioxidant called kaempferol, which is best known for its ability to ease inflammation. But that's not all. Some research says that eating foods high in kaempferol, like broccoli, is a great way to help reduce your risk for certain cancers.

Cabbage

The cheapest way to heal your gut

Good nutrition can seem tricky, especially when you want to save money on that ever-growing grocery bill. Why not try cabbage? It's an amazingly cheap and versatile vegetable that protects you against all sorts of major ailments that disturb the digestive system. From constipation to colorectal cancer, cabbage is a wise investment in health for only about 62 cents per pound.

Cabbage combats constipation. Oh, that taboo topic — constipation. This common condition affects up to 20% of adults. Fortunately, most people can get things moving again just by changing up what they're eating.

So add cabbage to your menu. It's high in H2O. And since dehydration can lead to constipation, munching on more water-packed foods is a no-brainer.

In addition, this leafy veggie is full of fiber. By bulking and softening your stool, fiber shortens the time it takes for food to travel through your digestive tract, keeping you regular. As a bonus, cabbage contains a special form of fiber called prebiotics. When your friendly gut bacteria feast on a buffet of prebiotics, they produce short-chain fatty acids. These fuel the cells that line the wall of your colon and help move things along.

Use your plate to ward off colorectal cancer. The American Cancer Society has some great news. Since the 1980s, rates of colon and rectal cancer diagnoses have gone down. Experts agree that one reason may be improved lifestyle changes, including healthier diets.

Scientists have a few theories about why cabbage may be the diet change you need. Because fiber moves stool along quickly, there's less time for cancer-causing chemicals to interact with your colon walls. Plus those short-chain fatty acids produced when fiber ferments in your gut may protect against cancer.

Cruciferous veggies like cabbage also contain nutrients called glucosinolates that may help destroy tumor cells. No wonder studies have shown that eating higher amounts of cabbage is linked to a lower risk of colorectal cancer.

Choose the kind of cabbage that offers red-hot heart perks

Cabbage has long had a humble reputation, but all that's about to change. Chefs and journalists alike have hailed this versatile veggie as "the new kale." And once you get a load of its benefits for your heart, you may be singing its praises, too.

Go red to love on your ticker. Red cabbage is packed with special nutrients called anthocyanins, making it both pretty and practical. These natural chemicals are responsible for the vegetable's vibrant color, and they acts as antioxidants. Researchers think that when it comes to combatting heart disease, antioxidants do their part by reducing inflammation and blood vessel damage.

If you're not convinced yet, maybe this will help. A recent review of studies found that people who regularly ate foods loaded with anthocyanins had a lower risk of heart disease. Another study of over 90,000 nurses found that young and middle-aged women who ate more anthocyanin-rich foods had a lower risk of heart attack. Bon appétit!

Put the pressure on high blood pressure. Anthocyanins are also linked to better blood pressure, but those aren't the only artery-loving nutrients cabbage has to offer. Just 1 cup of red cabbage takes care of 6% to 8% of your daily potassium needs.

Potassium helps your body get rid of sodium, a mineral known to hike blood pressure. It also helps by relaxing the walls of your blood vessels.

Colorful cabbage for clogged arteries. Want to try something new? How about dining on red and black cabbage, also known as lacinato kale? One intriguing study found that eating a 300-gram bag of red and black cabbage each day lowered total cholesterol, bad LDL cholesterol, and oxidized LDL — which may be the most harmful form of cholesterol. The researchers say benefits could be related to the fiber and other nutrients such as anthocyanins and carotenoids.

Chefs beware! Cooking red cabbage can lower the amounts of helpful anthocyanins and glucosinolates. Instead, try shredding it into a sassy raw salad or a crispy taco topping.

It's no shocker that fiber is involved. Studies have already shown that fiber helps your body whisk away excess cholesterol. And a crunchy cup of chopped cabbage has almost 2 grams of it. Every little bit helps in reaching the daily recommended 21 grams of fiber for senior women and 30 grams for older men.

 Bright idea

For centuries, people have used cabbage leaves as a folk remedy to ease painful joints. And now science backs them up.

One four-week study found that people with osteoarthritis in their knees got relief after applying cabbage leaves to the affected area for two hours a day. Want to give it a try? Here's how.

Place two or three outer cabbage leaves on a cutting board and remove the hard stems with a sharp knife. Gently roll a glass bottle or mason jar over the leaves to release some of their juices. Place the leaves on the front and back of your knee and cover with cling wrap. Then loosely bandage the area to keep the poultice in place.

Leave on for at least an hour. You can rewrap the knee later in the day using fresh cabbage leaves.

Cauliflower

Supercharge your health with sulforaphane

Cauliflower may not be as eye-catching as its bright green broccoli cousin, but it's loaded with good-for-you nutrients. One of the standout stars is sulforaphane.

This compound has antioxidant properties that reduce inflammation and the risk of these chronic health problems.

Kiss high blood pressure and clogged arteries goodbye. Cruciferous veggies like cauliflower are a heart-healthy choice thanks to the powerful anti-inflammatory and antioxidant activity of sulforaphane.

Inflammation is linked to high blood pressure, unhealthy cholesterol levels, and hardened arteries. In test tube and animal studies, sulforaphane extracts have reduced inflammation. And study authors suggest the nutrient may lend a hand in lowering blood pressure, improving levels of HDL or "good" cholesterol, and enhancing blood flow.

Keeping your blood pressure in the normal range and your arteries clear slashes your risk of stroke and heart attack.

Improve your blood sugar levels with a tasty alt. Besides an increased risk of type 2 diabetes, unhealthy blood sugar levels are linked to weight gain and problems with the heart, kidneys, and eyes.

One study showed that a daily sulforaphane extract over 12 weeks improved blood sugar levels in obese people with type 2 diabetes. The extract came from broccoli sprouts, but you don't have to wait for studies on cauliflower to start adding more of this sulforaphane-rich veggie to your meals.

Cauliflower is already a great substitute because it's low in carbohydrates, which raise your blood sugar. Eat it mashed as a yummy alternative to high-carb mashed potatoes. Or try it riced as an excellent stand-in for starchy white rice.

A delicious way to protect against cancer. Eating more fruits and vegetables is one way to defend yourself against cancer. Plant foods like cauliflower contain a wide spectrum of phytochemicals that keep carcinogens, or cancer-causing substances, from doing their dirty work.

In fact, in lab and animal studies, sulforaphane has proven powerful enough to disrupt the formation of new cancer cells and the spread of existing ones.

 Kitchen hacks

In side-by-side comparisons, researchers discovered that steaming cauliflower preserves more nutrients than boiling or blanching. Stir-frying and microwaving are also good bets for maximum nutrition.

Prep fresh cauliflower by picking off the green outer leaves and then cutting it into quarters. Carve off the core, and use a knife or your hands to break it into florets. People often throw out the stem and leaves, but you can use them to make homemade stock or finely chop them into soups or salads.

To steam, fill a pot with enough water to cover the bottom and bring the water to a simmer. Place the cauliflower in a steamer basket or stainless steel colander and set it into the pot. Cover your cauliflower and cook for about 10 minutes or until fork-tender.

Once steamed, you can season the cauliflower or mash it for a low-carb alternative to mashed potatoes.

The secret to younger-looking skin

Fine lines. Dryness. Thinning skin. Want to put the brakes on all that? It may be time to cut out some of those carbs and fats, then add a few helpings of vitamin C. Here's why.

Scientists analyzed the diets of more than 4,000 women and found that those who ate more carbohydrates and fatty foods had more wrinkles and thinner skin. On the other hand, eating more vitamin C-rich foods was associated with fewer wrinkles and less dryness.

Cauliflower fills the bill. It's low in fat and carbs. Plus 1 cup of raw cauliflower has 53 milligrams of vitamin C, which is more than half the amount you need in a day.

Vitamin C protects your skin in several ways, starting with its role in collagen synthesis. Collagen is a structural protein found in skin. Your body makes less of it with age, which contributes to wrinkles. But getting enough vitamin C helps your body make collagen.

Acting as an antioxidant, vitamin C also helps defend against the sun's damaging ultraviolet rays — a leading cause of aging skin, age spots, and skin cancer. And as an added bonus, the sulforaphane in cauliflower offers even more antioxidant protection.

Crunch on cauliflower for better brainpower

Cauliflower has a brain-boosting nutrient that you've probably never heard of. What is this underappreciated powerhouse? Choline.

Many people don't get enough of this essential nutrient. Maybe that's because the amount most people eat is not up to snuff with how much the body needs — 550 milligrams (mg) for men and 425 mg for women.

Don't slack off. Choline plays a role in maintaining cell membranes and helps your cells signal to each other — a VIP job in the brain and nervous system, aka your body's command center. What's more, several studies have linked getting plenty of choline with better brain function.

- In a Norwegian study, scientists compared choline blood levels from over 2,000 men and women in their 70s with their performance on a series of cognitive tests. Those with low levels of choline scored worse on tests involving motor skills, visual perception, and working memory compared to those with high levels of choline.

- In another study, scientists assessed choline intake from food questionnaires completed by nearly 1,400 men and women with an average age of 60. Those who ate the most choline-rich foods performed better on verbal and visual memory tests than those who ate the least. In addition, early higher choline intake was linked to smaller patchy areas in the brain, which are believed to be a sign of blood vessel disease and could signal a higher risk of stoke and dementia.

Luckily, cooked cauliflower gets you started off on the right foot with 60 mg of choline per cup. Combine it with other high-choline foods like beef, soybeans, and chicken.

 Watch out

No doubt, cauliflower is one healthy veggie, but it doesn't agree with everyone. Cauliflower and other cruciferous veggies are known for making people gassy. It's a high-FODMAP food, meaning it contains a group of carbohydrates that can be hard to digest and trigger gas, bloating, and constipation in some people.

For those struggling with irritable bowel syndrome (IBS), these side effects can be especially troubling. IBS sufferers often find relief on a low-FODMAP diet. So if you're sensitive to FODMAPs or follow a low-FODMAP diet, you may have to pass on cauliflower.

The same goes for those who take blood thinner medication to manage a heart condition. That's because cauliflower contains vitamin K, which can make some blood thinners less effective. While taking these meds, decide with your doctor how much vitamin K you'll eat daily. Then avoid changing that amount.

Eggplant

4 reasons you should start eating this Mediterranean staple today

When was the last time you had a helping of aubergine? What about a serving of brinjal? Never? Perhaps you know this delicious cuisine by its common name — eggplant.

This food is a staple of the Mediterranean diet, a meal plan linked to a reduced risk of heart disease, weight gain, diabetes, cancer, and Alzheimer's. The diet is high in fruits, veggies, whole grains, and a whole host of delicious foods you probably already eat. But if you've been neglecting eggplant, you're missing out on the chance to double up on these health benefits.

While eggplants are commonly used as vegetables in dishes, they are considered fruits based on how they grow. They come from a flowering plant and also contain seeds and pulp, which makes them berries botanically. No matter what you call them, they're delicious combined with garlic, peppers, onions, tomatoes, and more.

Sup your way to a slimmer body. Internet stars on YouTube may tout the slimming benefits of eggplant water, but drinking the aftermath of boiled brinjal isn't proven to help anyone drop the pounds.

However, incorporating eggplants into your recipes could help you lose weight, thanks to fiber. This nutrient keeps your belly full, so you avoid overindulging. One cup of cubed eggplant packs a generous 2.5 grams of fiber and has only 20.5 calories.

Since eggplants are a naturally low-cal food, they make it easier to stay within your calorie needs and watch those pounds drop. So stir-fry or grill them as a savory alternative for high-calorie, no-fiber meats.

A happy choice for your ticker and taste buds. The same fiber that keeps you full, also helps lower cholesterol, say experts. Maintaining healthy cholesterol levels keeps a sticky substance called plaque from building up in your arteries. Too much plaque buildup increases your risk of artery blockage, which can lead to heart problems.

Eggplants are also rich in other heart-healthy nutrients, like the neurotransmitter acetylcholine. That's the ingredient Japanese researchers say may be responsible for the results of their recent study — the first evidence that eggplant may lower blood pressure in people.

For 12 weeks, a group of stressed participants took a daily dose of a placebo or eggplant powder made from about 1/3 cup of fresh eggplant. Eating eggplant improved blood pressure, compared to taking the placebo. That's great news since lowering blood pressure helps ease the burden on your pumping heart so it doesn't have to work as hard.

Keep a tight rein on your blood sugar. If you have diabetes, keeping your blood sugar levels stable is a must. How can eggplant help you beat blood sugar spikes? Fiber to the rescue again. It helps your body absorb sugar more slowly, which can stop those dreaded energy spikes and crashes.

Early studies have also identified powerful phytochemicals in purple, white, and graffiti eggplants. Scientists believe these nutrients have the potential to delay the absorption of carbs, keeping glucose levels balanced.

Fight free radicals to shore up your defenses. Antioxidants — it might be a marketing buzzword, but scientists think these substances may have the clout to back some of the hype. They protect your body by neutralizing harmful free radicals. Those are unstable atoms that steal electrons from other molecules, causing damage and contributing to chronic diseases.

Eggplants are just loaded with antioxidants, particularly an anthocyanin called nasunin. Test tube and animal studies show these antioxidants protect cells from DNA damage, fight inflammation, and combat cancer cells.

Nasunin, the main antioxidant in eggplants, is what gives the fruits their purple color. So no surprise, you have to eat the peel to get the benefits. The skin of larger eggplants can be tough, though. For the tastiest results, buy small eggplants with thin, more tender skin, and enjoy them braised or sauteed.

Get your fill by eating eggplants regularly along with other high-antioxidant foods found in the Mediterranean diet, like berries, nuts, and leafy greens.

✕ Kitchen hacks

When shopping for eggplant, look for ones with smooth, glossy skin as a sign of freshness. They should be slightly firm to the touch, but not hard. If you push down on the eggplant and the skin punctures, it's too ripe and not of the best quality. You'll also want to look for a green stem to signify prime ripeness.

For best results when preparing eggplant, slice it first and salt liberally. Let the eggplant sit for an hour or so before draining the juice. Then rinse and pat dry the slices. All this draws out the compound solanine, which can cause eggplants to taste bitter. It will also keep them from turning mushy.

Eggplant can be prepared in several ways, including roasted and mashed into baba ganoush, a traditional Arabic eggplant dip. It's also good baked, sauteed, or mixed into a vegetable stew.

Garlic

3 'hearty' reasons to make this bulb a staple in your kitchen

Someone dies from heart disease every 36 seconds in the United States, according to the Centers for Disease Control and Prevention. No mincing words — this disease is a heartbreaking problem. It robs many people of their lives way too early with devastating experiences like heart attack and stroke.

The good news is you have some control over heart disease — starting with your plate. And one of the front-runners for heart protection is garlic. It's the amazing natural antibiotic that takes care of your ticker in three powerful ways.

Crush cholesterol with flavorful fare. Cholesterol gets a bad rap in the heart health world, but it's not really something to be afraid of. It's a normal fat that everyone needs for many body functions, like making hormones and vitamin D. It's so important that your liver can miraculously produce all the cholesterol your body needs.

But like anything else, when cholesterol is too high, things can go wonky. Not to fear, garlic is here.

An analysis published in the journal *Nutrition Reviews* evaluated 39 studies on garlic powder, aged garlic extract, garlic oil, or raw garlic. It showed

How about a little citrus on the side? It goes great with garlic. Plus one study showed that a daily combo of 1 tablespoon of lemon juice and 20 grams of raw garlic — equal to almost seven cloves — helped lower cholesterol. That was compared to having each individually or none at all for eight weeks.

that when participants with high cholesterol took garlic for more than two months, total cholesterol levels dropped an average of 8%.

Supplements that protect your arteries. High blood pressure, aka hypertension, can lead to hardened, thickened arteries. This isn't safe because the damage may eventually block blood flow to the heart. Scientists are scrambling to find hypertension help, and it looks like garlic is promising.

In fact, a review of studies involving over 500 people showed that garlic supplements can improve hypertension. Most of the studies used 600 to 900 milligrams (mg) of garlic powder or 1,200 mg of aged garlic extract each day. Study authors say the drop in blood pressure is associated with a 16% to 40% lower risk of heart disease.

 Kitchen hacks

Every chef seems to have their favorite way to peel garlic, but here are two reliable methods that don't require fancy tools.

Use the knife technique to smash and peel. It works even better if you chop off the root end before you begin.

1. Separate a clove from the bulb and lay it on your cutting board.

2. Place the flat side of a chef's knife on the bulb.

3. Rocking the knife, press carefully, just firmly enough to separate the skin from the clove without crushing it.

4. Voila! Peel it easy-peasy.

Try the hot water hack. It's great if you're leaving the cloves whole since there's no risk of crushing them.

1. In a small bowl, soak unpeeled cloves in very hot water for one minute.

2. Now that the skin is loose, simply peel it away.

Break up stroke-causing blockages. Blood clots are a danger-ous problem. When a blood clot blocks the way to your heart or brain, it can lead to a heart attack or stroke. Compounds in garlic are thought to stop blood from clumping, which means the veggie could help your blood flow more smoothly.

Because of this blood-thinning effect, it's important to tell your doctor before eating lots of garlic or taking supplements. Both could interfere with certain medications and may not be safe for people who have a bleeding disorder or need surgery.

Get to the root of joint and bone bothers

Strictly speaking, garlic is a root vegetable. But your body won't complain if you call it an herb or spice, so long as you're getting plenty of it. That's because there's a link between this bold bulb and joint and bone health.

A natural way to relieve joint pain. Osteoarthritis is a painful joint condition characterized by a breakdown of cartilage. Garlic has an anti-inflammatory effect that may offer some relief.

In one study, overweight women with knee osteoarthritis took 1,000 milligrams of garlic tablets or a placebo each day for 12 weeks. Pain scores and levels of a hormone linked to inflamma-tion dropped in the garlic group but not the placebo group.

In another study, researchers found that women who ate more allium vegetables — like garlic, onions, shallots, chives, and leeks — were less likely to suffer from hip osteoarthritis. They think a compound in garlic called diallyl disulfide limits cartilage-damaging enzymes.

"While we don't yet know if eating garlic will lead to high levels of this component in the joint, these findings may point the way toward future treatments and prevention of hip osteoarthritis," says lead author Frances Williams, Ph.D., of King's College London.

Support for your skeleton. Bones are often out of sight and out of mind — until one breaks. Unfortunately, bone fractures are common, especially for postmenopausal women. Researchers say roughly 4 out of 10 white women over the age of 50 will experience a hip, spine, or wrist fracture. What's a girl to do?

Well, scientists think that bone loss after menopause is related to reduced hormone levels for women. And garlic supplementation seems to help keep estrogen elevated and minimize bone loss, at least in animal studies.

Research on small groups of postmenopausal women with osteoporosis is encouraging. The studies showed that garlic supplements may have a beneficial effect on markers of inflammation and oxidative stress, two factors linked to brittle bones.

 Bright idea

Have a green thumb? Consider adding garlic to your garden to reap big rewards.

First off, garlic is a good choice for companion gardening. This is a fancy name for the centuries-old method of growing crops together so they benefit from each other.

- Bug buffer. Planting garlic between strawberry rows may keep spider mites from destroying your juicy, red fruit. Avid gardeners also plant these aromatic herbs beside lettuce to fend off aphids.

- Soil saver. Growing peppers and garlic together can improve the soil by increasing important nutrients. Same goes for planting it with cucumbers or eggplant.

Finally, your efforts will earn the bonus harvest of garlic scapes. These curly stems sprout from hardneck garlic about one month before bulb harvest time, and trimming them will encourage robust clove growth. Cut each scape at the base after it forms a spiral at the top. Then chop them finely for a sauteed sauce or pesto. Yum!

Ginger-garlic greatness: Tasty combos with 2 punchy perks

Nutty garlic and zesty, sweet ginger. Mmm, a delicious duo. But they do more than tickle your taste buds. Both contain nutrients that may help you skirt some unsavory conditions. Fuse them with powerful ingredients in these signature dishes for an all-out fortifying feast.

Cut your odds of cancer with veggie tikka masala. This flavorful Indian combo of marinated vegetables in a spiced curry sauce is a showstopper at dinnertime.

But you probably care more about what it may stop in your body — cancer. A great deal of that protection comes from garlic and onions, two allium vegetables that know how to bring the fight.

Researchers have been aware of the link between alliums and cancer for years. And now a recent study has examined the allium-eating habits of more than 1,500 adults with and without colorectal cancer.

"There seems to be a trend," says senior author Dr. Zhi Li, of the First Hospital of China Medical University. "The greater the amount of allium vegetables, the better the protection."

Participants who saw the most protection ate about 74 grams of alliums a day. You could get about a third of that in a serving of veggie tikka masala.

But that's not all. This dish also contains ginger and turmeric. Good news since extracts of both have demonstrated cancer-fighting activity, alone and in a mixture with — you guessed it — garlic.

The brains behind garlic-ginger chili sauce. This savory sauce goes great with Chinese-style chicken, rice, or noodles. The tasty trio of garlic, ginger, and chili peppers makes for a star-studded cast, but garlic takes center stage.

That's according to recent animal research presented at an American Physiological Society conference. Results revealed that a compound found in this bulb may help offset age-related gut changes linked to memory problems.

"Our findings suggest that dietary administration of garlic containing allyl sulfide could help maintain healthy gut microorganisms and improve cognitive health in the elderly," says study co-leader Jyotirmaya Behera, Ph.D., of the University of Louisville.

It's too early to say how much garlic might do the trick. But adding this super sauce to your arsenal seems like a no-brainer. Especially since previous research agrees that garlic might give your memory an edge. Not to mention animal studies suggest that ginger and chili peppers may also support the noggin.

Banishing garlic breath:
How to fend off the funk

Enjoying garlic tends to have a stinky side effect — halitosis, more commonly known as bad breath. Unfortunately, the smell isn't limited to your mouth. It permeates from your lungs hours after you eat garlic. This means the odor will linger even after brushing your teeth. Phew!

Not to worry. You can graze on garlic without the lingering evidence. A study showed that people who ate garlic with raw apples, lettuce, or mint leaves had much milder breath than those who ate garlic alone.

Scientists think these foods contain chemicals that neutralize offending odors in garlic. So keep yourself kissable. Consider pairing an apple-romaine salad with your garlic-marinated salmon.

A closer look
Juicing

When it comes to eating fruits and veggies, more is always better. Still, it can be tough meeting the American Heart Association's recommendation of four to five daily servings of each. Sure sounds like a lot of chewing.

Enter juicing. It's the process of squeezing, grating, and pressing fruits and vegetables until the liquid is extracted from the fleshy part. Most folks nowadays use a machine for this, with the juice pouring out of a spout while the fibrous pulp remains behind.

Drinking fresh juice shouldn't be confused with having a smoothie, which is made by pureeing whole pieces of produce in a blender. Lots of people add milk, yogurt, crushed ice, nuts, or seeds to the liquid and pulp mixture, which produces a thick, creamy drink.

But let's get back to juicing and the million-dollar question. Is this trendy process all it's cracked up to be? Read on for the benefits and how to easily correct the drawbacks.

Fiber is key. Juicing is a great way to provide your body with plant-based vitamins and minerals that you miss if you don't eat enough produce. But, when you juice a fruit or vegetable, you remove all the tummy-filling fiber that helps to lower cholesterol and keep your digestive tract running smoothly.

The fix? Don't throw away the pulp that's left sitting in your juicer. Instead, blend some in with your drink. Aside from the health benefits, leftover fruit mash also adds moisture, texture, and a burst of flavor to muffin and pancake batter. And the vegetable kind goes great in soups, sauces, dips, and casseroles.

You can mix either kind of pulp with reduced-fat cream cheese for a tasty spread on crackers and sandwiches.

Watch the sugar. Of course, any 100% natural juice that you prepare in the kitchen is going to have more nutrients than sugar-sweetened soda. But when you juice fruits like oranges, apples, and pomegranates, you get all their natural sweetness in concentrated amounts. That can mean winding up with lots of sugar and unexpected calories in a small amount of liquid.

The answer? Pour a small portion of fruit juice in your cup and then fill it to the brim with club soda. You'll get the sweet taste with less sugar. Or you can focus your juicing on veggies like celery, cucumbers, parsley, kale, spinach, and Swiss chard. Then add just a little bit of fruit as a sweetener. Either way, your waistline — and blood glucose levels — will thank you.

Now for the inside scoop on juicing safely.

- Wash all fruits and veggies thoroughly, even if you're going to peel them. The same goes for pre-cut produce, which is more likely to harbor bacteria.

- Drink your juice immediately after making it. Otherwise, light and air will destroy many of the nutrients. This will also prevent harmful germs from getting a chance to grow in it. After all, homemade juice isn't pasteurized.

- Don't rely only on juicing to lose weight quickly. Instead, include fresh juice as part of a healthy diet that includes lean protein, whole grains, low-fat dairy, and whole fruits and veggies.

Of course, one of the joys of making your own juice is knowing exactly what is in it. But sometimes you just don't have the time for all the slicing and dicing.

So if you're looking for fresh juice at the supermarket, ensure you get the healthiest kind by choosing one that contains only fruits, vegetables, and possibly water.

Avoid any that have added sugars, flavorings, or artificial sweeteners. And opt for pasteurized juices as they are less likely to cause a foodborne illness.

Greens

Food for thought — 2 ways to maintain your brain

Here's something you'll definitely want to keep in "MIND." Scientists have developed an eating plan specifically designed to support brain health. Sticking to the MIND diet can help you build a wall against mental decline and Alzheimer's disease.

The MIND menu — a hybrid of the Mediterranean and DASH diets — focuses on plant-based fare like leafy greens, whole grains, fruits, nuts, berries, beans, and olive oil. This mix of delicious foods is rich in antioxidants, compounds that can prevent rogue molecules from damaging brain cells. Plus, they help fend off heart disease and diabetes, two risk factors for developing Alzheimer's disease.

In effect, keeping your brain healthy can be as simple as going to the garden or your fresh produce aisle. Just keep your eyes peeled for an incredible plant — leafy greens. Two nutrients in these important veggies are especially beneficial for a tiptop noggin.

The Dietary Approaches to Stop Hypertension (DASH) diet has been around for decades — and for good reason. It's the most efficient and effective way to lower your blood pressure, cholesterol, and heart attack risk. The plan features lots of fiber, limits salt and saturated fats, and emphasizes foods rich in heart-healthy magnesium and potassium. No medication necessary!

Folate keeps 2 at bay. You won't believe how vital this B vitamin is to keeping you sharp as a tack. Research has found an association between seniors deficient in folate and an increased risk of developing dementia. How much higher? A whopping 3.5 times more likely to get the disease.

And while you can choose among hundreds of varieties of greens, it may be as simple as focusing on two — spinach and escarole. Just 1 cup of cooked spinach contains an incredible 263 micrograms (mcg) of this B vitamin, more than half of the recommended daily amount. Add a cup of cooked escarole — a curly green that loses some of its bitterness as it cooks — and you'll get another 103 mcg. Not too shabby if you're looking to have a sharp brain at 70!

Lutein stops your brain from aging. Your body can't produce this antioxidant on its own, so make sure you're eating plenty of leafy greens to get enough. A study from the University of Illinois found that young to middle-aged adults who ate more lutein-rich foods had neural responses in their brains that were more on par with younger folks than with their peers. More studies are needed to find out why, so stay tuned.

Greens high in lutein include kale, romaine lettuce, and spinach. You can easily get more of them in your diet by sauteing, steaming, or adding them to soups. They all go great in smoothies and salads, and as a nutritious wrap in place of tortillas or bread.

5 leafy greens you're not eating but should be

Leafy greens are packed with nutrients that help improve your health in so many ways. It's a good idea to be adventurous when choosing the greens on your plate because each variety contains different amounts of potent plant compounds that protect your eyes, bones, brain, colon, and more. Here are five delicious greens to try.

Arugula. People usually eat this veggie raw on sandwiches or as a base for a salad, but you can also cook it. With its bold, peppery taste and delicate texture, arugula is prized by chefs for adding a tart and pleasantly bitter component to dishes like gourmet pizza or pasta dishes. It's also a good source of vitamin K.

Chard. This easy-to-grow vegetable is tasty as a side dish or cooked into soup. Chard varieties such as Swiss or rainbow are incredibly delicious sauteed with garlic and splashed with vinegar or lemon juice. Eat a cup of cooked Swiss chard for 477% to 636% of the vitamin K you need each day, along with lots of fiber, iron, potassium, vitamin C, magnesium, and vitamin E.

Bok choy. A type of Chinese cabbage, bok choy is a unique mild-tasting vegetable that is perfect as a tender-crisp addition to stir-fry with notes of garlic and ginger. This fantastic vegetable contains lots of flavonols that help fight cancer-causing free radicals, and it's also full of vitamins C, K, and A.

> Here's some good news. Frozen veggies — including greens — have just as much nutritional value as fresh. So keep a few bags of kale, collards, and spinach in your freezer. Take them straight to the stovetop when you're ready to cook. No washing, chopping, or defrosting necessary.

Mustard greens. These greens are delicious sauteed or served with white beans in a stew. They have a bold, spicy flavor you will love as much as the powerful nutrients they provide. In addition to fiber and vitamins E, K, and C, you'll score 96% to 124% of your daily vitamin A with 1 cup of cooked mustard greens.

Turnip greens. Chop them off the top of your turnips, then rinse and cook them as you would any other green. They have a zesty, peppery bite and work well in comfort foods such as casseroles and hearty soups. A cup of cooked turnip greens provides 44% to 53% of your daily recommended vitamin C, plus plenty of fiber, calcium, and vitamins K, A, and E.

Bright idea

Have you ever felt like your teeth were covered in carpet after eating spinach? You're not imagining things. Two components in spinach, oxalic acid and calcium, react when you chew, causing them to combine to form calcium oxalate. This new substance takes the form of tiny crystals, which feel rough and fuzzy, sometimes even sticky, on the surface of your teeth. You have solutions.

First, if you gently steam your spinach, it may prevent this grainy texture from developing. Secondly, if you squeeze a bit of zesty lemon juice on your spinach, the vitamin C may help dissolve oxalic acid, leaving your teeth free of fuzz. Luckily, a splash of lemon is delicious on steamed spinach, so give this technique a try for smooth, clean teeth.

Superstar spinach enhances your health from head to toe

An exceptional nutrient lineup is how spinach earned the coveted superfood title. It sports these amazing health benefits, and it tastes great, too.

Keep your bones solid and fracture-free. Bone breaks and osteoporosis are an increasing risk as you get older, especially for women. In fact, about half of ladies over 50 will break a bone in their lifetime. Both osteoporosis and fractures are linked to not getting enough vitamin K.

This nutrient helps proteins in your body that are responsible for forming and strengthening bones. And a cup of cooked spinach sweeps the board with 741% to 988% of the K you need each day.

Cut your risk of colon cancer. According to the Centers for Disease Control and Prevention, colorectal cancer is the second deadliest cancer in the United States. New animal research suggests that spinach may help block the growth of colon polyps, which are clumps of cells lining the colon that can turn into potentially fatal cancer.

Spinach contains antioxidants such as chlorophyll, which fight against cancer-causing free radicals. These greens also support a healthy gut microbiome, meaning they help keep your colon in a thriving, cancer-resistant state.

Magnesium balances your moods. This vital mineral plays an essential role in brain chemistry, including how mood-regulating neurotransmitters do their jobs. Magnesium deficiencies are associated with depression, agitation, confusion, anxiety, and delirium. One cup of cooked spinach contains about half of your daily needs.

Your waistline will thank you for eating spinach. Promising research on spinach extract shows it could help blast belly fat by reducing your appetite. A small study found that structures in spinach membranes called thylakoids can banish hunger and cravings — even for tempting foods like sweet and salty snacks. Thylakoids also helped overweight participants in another study to feel more satisfied compared to a placebo.

Lutein in greens protects your peepers. Spinach can boost your eye health with a nutrient called lutein. This inflammation-busting antioxidant has been shown to help prevent cataracts and macular degeneration — diseases that can lead to severe vision loss. Your body can't make lutein, so get it through your diet in foods like spinach and other leafy greens.

Banish bad cholesterol with lutein-packed spinach. Lutein plays another role in promoting good health, making spinach an even more attractive addition to your plate. In one study, this powerful pigment reduced dangerous LDL cholesterol levels and triglycerides, as well as markers of inflammation, in people with a type of hardening of the arteries called atherosclerosis.

 Boost the benefits

Spice up your boring salad by choosing a tastier, more interesting base. Throw in some kale, arugula, radicchio, dandelion, or watercress. These vibrantly colored greens will tantalize your taste buds, and they're a lot more nutritionally dense than the go-to salad staple — iceberg lettuce.

Collards: A delicious down-home vegetable to keep your arteries clear

Collard greens are loaded with a powerful vitamin that neutralizes artery-clogging toxins. While they're packed with many healthful vitamins and minerals, it's the B vitamins, namely B6 and folate, that show your heart some love.

Vitamin B6 is responsible for many important jobs in your body, including breaking down the carbohydrates and fats you eat. Folate is associated with a reduced risk of chronic diseases, like cardiovascular disease and several cancers. Both B6 and folate are water-soluble, meaning they can't be stored. Any extra you consume will be flushed out, and you must replace them each day.

A large study on nearly 60,000 people showed that getting more of these two powerhouse vitamins is linked to a lower risk of death from heart failure in men and from stroke, heart disease, and cardiovascular disease in women. This effect may be due to vitamin B6 and folate lowering the levels of an amino acid called homocysteine by breaking it down. High amounts of homocysteine may damage the lining of your arteries and cause blood clots.

Getting enough of these vital B vitamins will help you reap the benefits. Collard greens are an excellent and delicious way to shore up your stores of B6 and folate. Women over age 50 should aim to get 1.5 milligrams (mg) of vitamin B6 each day, while senior men need 1.7 mg. For folate, the goal is 400 micrograms (mcg) daily.

A one-cup serving of cooked collard greens contains 0.2 mg of vitamin B6, about 13% to 15% of your daily recommended amount. The same serving size contains 135 mcg of folate — about 34% of your daily needs. That's a pretty big nutritional punch for a side dish.

Other appetizing sources of these B vitamins include leafy greens like spinach and kale, whole grains, fish, liver, meat, and fortified cereals. So fill your plate with these delectable foods, including a side of collard greens for clear arteries and a healthy heart.

Vitamin K-rich greens could save your life

It might seem like a bold statement, but science says eating your greens could save your life. Low levels of vitamin K1, also known as phylloquinone, are associated with a higher risk of death.

Research published in *The American Journal of Clinical Nutrition* studied 3,891 participants with an average age of 65 and found that those who had lower levels of vitamin K1 circulating in their bloodstreams had a 19% increased risk of dying from any cause within the next 13 years or so compared to those who had enough K1. Vitamin K aids proteins that keep calcium from building up in your arteries, known as calcification.

"Similar to when a rubber band dries out and loses its elasticity, when veins and arteries are calcified, blood pumps less efficiently, causing a variety of complications," says Dr. Daniel Weiner, a nephrologist at Tufts Medical Center and one of the study authors.

As you may have guessed, the foods highest in this lifesaving nutrient are greens. In fact, a cup of cooked spinach, Swiss chard, kale, collards, beet greens, and turnip greens each contain more than 400% of the recommended daily value of 90 micrograms (mcg) for women and 120 mcg for men.

Cooking your greens helps concentrate the amount of vitamin K you get in a cup, but eating them raw is also an excellent way of reaching your daily amount. You can chop them into salads, steam them, and add them to stir-fries, soups, or eggs.

 Kitchen hacks

Greens are delicious and healthy, but they can spoil quickly if not stored correctly. After bringing your greens home or in from the garden, wash them gently with cool water. Next, dry them with paper towels delicately, so you don't bruise them. If your greens have large leaves, you can tear them into smaller pieces.

Store washed and dried greens in a plastic zip-top bag lined with a clean paper towel. The paper towel will absorb the remaining moisture to prevent sogginess and rot. Press the air out of the bag before sealing, and put it in your fridge's crisper section. If you have too many greens for a bag, use the same method with a sealable plastic container. Using this method, you can preserve your greens for up to a week.

Onions

Beneficial bulbs layer on 3 powerful perks

The Queen threatened to behead the Seven of Spades for bringing the cook tulip roots instead of onions in Lewis Carroll's *Alice's Adventures in Wonderland*. A major faux pas to be sure. After all tulips don't contain inulin, the natural fiber you need lots of, but have probably never heard of. Here's why you, too, will be demanding your fair share of onions.

Keep your gut happy and healthy. When you eat onions, you're not just feeding yourself. You're also feeding the good bacteria in your gut. That's because the inulin found in the veggie is a type of prebiotic.

This fiber is a favorite food of the friendly bacteria in your gut and helps them thrive. In fact, a recent review of studies found that taking 5 to 20 grams of inulin supplements daily improved the abundance of several species of good gut bacteria.

Get 5 grams of inulin when you eat about one medium-sized raw onion or almost two medium-sized cooked onions. You'll be glad you did because good bugs help crowd out bad bacteria, which improves digestion and helps keep you regular.

Give calcium a helping hand. Along with getting enough calcium and vitamin D in your diet, inulin may be the secret weapon to building stronger bones. A firm frame is essential for preventing fractures and staying active throughout life.

Luckily, digesting inulin creates short-chain fatty acids that lower the pH of your intestines, making it easier for your body to absorb bone-building calcium. Not only that, inulin encourages certain proteins to soak up more calcium from your gut.

Just how much should you aim for? A brand-new review says that taking 8 to 10 grams of inulin supplements daily long term may improve calcium absorption in adults.

Boost weight loss with a special fiber. Looking to shed a few pounds? Make sure onions are a part of your plan to slim down. Scientists think the inulin in them helps control appetite.

They tested out the theory in a small group of adults with pre-diabetes. Participants took either 30 grams of inulin or a cellulose supplement for 18 weeks. For the first nine weeks of the study, all participants went through a weight loss program with a dietitian. Then they continued taking the inulin or cellulose for nine more weeks with no support.

Though both groups had similar weight loss in the first half of the study, the biggest changes were seen in the second half. Those who took inulin lost an average of 3.7 more pounds.

You don't have to overindulge in onions, though. To get more inulin, also eat garlic, leeks, Jerusalem artichokes, asparagus, chicory roots, and dandelion greens.

 Bright idea

Give your onions a second life. If you accidentally leave them out too long and notice that they've sprouted, replant them to grow up to three new bulbs.

First, remove the papery skin of your onion. Next, peel or cut away the layers until you're left with the baby sprouts and the center of the bulb, including the base where the roots will grow.

Separate your sprouts, and place each little shoot into a glass of water. When white roots begin to grow, plant them in soil and wait three to four months before harvesting.

A trio of nutrients take onions from ho-hum to humdinger

Onions may not be too impressive at first glance, but this veggie is secretly an amazing superfood. And it's all due to three powerful nutrients.

Nourish your noggin with quercetin. While onions may grow underground, you don't have to be in the dark about how they can benefit your brain. Those powerful bulbs contain quercetin, an antioxidant that new research shows may protect against age-related cognitive decline.

In the study, a small group of Japanese adults, age 60 to 79, took either quercetin-rich onion powder or a placebo for 24 weeks. The group that took the antioxidant-packed onions scored better on tests measuring brain function.

The quercetin-rich onion powder amounted to about half of a medium-sized onion a day. If you want to try it out, make sure you choose the right variety. The researchers used white onion powder as a placebo since that kind is low in quercetin. Yellow and red onions contain much more of the nutrient.

Allicin protects against an assortment of ailments. Allicin is one of the eye-watering sulfur compounds released from freshly cut onions as a defense mechanism against pests. Science shows that it also helps defend against several conditions.

- A growing body of evidence suggests that allicin has anti-tumor activity. It may work by blocking the growth and spread of cancer cells.

- Allicin fights the bacteria *Helicobacter pylori*, a source of peptic ulcers. In a review of studies, allicin supplements as an add-on therapy increased the healing rate and remission of peptic ulcers and got rid of *H. pylori* faster than controls.

- Animal studies suggest allicin could help lower blood pressure, cholesterol, and inflammation in blood vessels.

Anthocyanins pack extra antioxidant power. Not only do red onions contain quercetin and allicin, they also have anthocyanins that give them their vibrant color.

Abdulmonem Murayyan, Ph.D. student and lead author of a study on the cancer-fighting power of onions, says anthocyanins may enhance the protective antioxidant activity of quercetin. The investigation, published in *Food Research International*, involved putting onion extracts onto colon cancer cells.

"We found onions are excellent at killing cancer cells," says Murayyan. "Onions activate pathways that encourage cancer cells to undergo cell death. They promote an unfavorable environment for cancer cells and they disrupt communication between cancer cells, which inhibits growth."

Human trials are next, but for now enjoy a mix of onion varieties to get a smorgasbord of nutrients.

 Kitchen hacks

Onions can make you cry because they release special enzymes when you slice and dice them. These enzymes produce sulfur gases, which cause stinging or burning sensations in your eyes. To keep from tearing up, try these clever tricks.

- Place your onions in the refrigerator for 30 minutes before you chop them. The cooler temperature slows the release of sulfur gases, so less of it reaches your eyes.

- Use a sharp knife. A dull one will damage more of the onion's cells, causing them to release more of the sulfur gases that make your eyes sting.

- If you're especially sensitive, invest in onion goggles to shield your eyes. Or use whatever you have on hand, like swim goggles or safety glasses.

Peppers

Add spice to your life — and health — with cayenne

Hot, spicy, and zesty are just a few of the words used to describe chili peppers. And capsaicin, pronounced cap-SAY-sin, is the natural substance that gives them their heat. But this compound does a lot more than simply ratchet up the flavor of worldwide cuisine.

People apply creams and gels containing capsaicin to soothe achy joints and muscles and to treat psoriasis, a skin disorder marked by itchy, scaly patches. Folks also use capsaicin-based nasal sprays to free up congestion. But it's downright remarkable what this substance does when eaten — it combats poor circulation and blood sugar spikes. Here's what else it does.

Shrink belly fat and reduce hunger with capsaicin. In one study, 80 overweight or obese adults took either a capsaicin extract or a placebo daily over 12 weeks. At the end of the study, those who took the supplement lost more belly fat than those who didn't. Researchers believe the capsaicin helped the participants to oxidize their fat.

Aren't interested in extracts? Then go straight to the source. Sprinkle a bit of cayenne pepper in your tomato juice and drink it 30 minutes before eating. According to Dutch researchers, folks who did this ate fewer calories yet felt more satisfied than a control group.

This compound helps to burn calories. There's good reason some like it hot. That's what scientists learned after giving capsaicin extracts to healthy adults over three months. At the end of that time, the participants lost more body fat than a control group that received a placebo.

So what happened? For starters, the folks who took the supplement reported a drop in appetite. That led them to decrease their calorie intake. The researchers also believe that capsaicin helps to boost the body's metabolism — the rate at which it burns calories. That, in turn, makes it easier to lose weight.

 Kitchen hacks

Love the taste and color of chili peppers but can't stand the heat? These pointers will help keep things cool in the kitchen.

The highest levels of capsaicin, the compound responsible for the burning sensation, are found in the chili's white membrane and seeds. So your best bet is to carve them out with a spoon. Scraping off the innermost layer of flesh will also help. Just be sure to wear gloves because capsaicin can irritate your skin. And keep your hands away from your face — particularly your eyes and mouth — when working with these peppers.

Here's another hack. Don't add your chilis when you begin to simmer food. Wait a while because cooking intensifies their spiciness. When you do mix in the hot peppers, use half the amount called for in the recipe. Taste as you go, adding more in small amounts until your food tastes just right.

Target high cholesterol with peppers. Hard to believe, but capsaicin doesn't just target body fat — it even lowers fats in the blood. And that's super important because high cholesterol is a major risk factor for clogged arteries, which can lead to heart attack and stroke.

Now for the good news. A review of nearly a dozen studies on the subject found that people who supplemented their diets with capsaicin saw improvements in their total cholesterol levels. Not only that, their levels of LDL, or "bad" cholesterol, were significantly lower than those of the people in the control group.

So why not reap the benefits of this compound by dusting some cayenne pepper over your next meal. For extra flavor, season your scrambled eggs, soups, and veggies with it. This zesty spice goes great on popcorn, trail mix, and nuts. You can even add it to plain yogurt for a healthy and delicious dip.

 Bright idea

Cayenne pepper is commonly used to give chili its "kick." But it can also give the boot to some unwanted insects and rodents taking up residence inside and outside your home. Savvy folks have long used this hot pepper to discourage everything from garden trespassers to kitchen invaders.

The simplest way to avoid pests in your garden is to sprinkle cayenne powder directly on and around the plants you're trying to protect. A mere 1/4 cup is probably all you'll need for a small garden. You can also do this in areas of the home or garage where you've seen mice pellets.

This spice shouldn't be harmful to any of your plants. But try it on a few leaves first and wait a day just to make sure. Wash your hands thoroughly after using cayenne powder. Same goes for your fruits and veggies before eating them.

Hot stuff: Here's to living longer and better

Heart disease and Alzheimer's are among the leading causes of death in the U.S. But it doesn't have to be that way. Research points to a small diet change that may help reduce the risk of both — the regular consumption of chili peppers.

Keep your ticker in tiptop shape. Italian researchers wanted to better understand the risk factors of death from chronic conditions.

So they looked at data on the eating habits of nearly 23,000 men and women who had been part of a study for years.

One team specifically examined the information to find out if eating hot peppers on a regular basis would have any effect on heart health. Turns out that people who ate chili peppers more than four times per week had a 34% lower risk of dying from cardiovascular disease than those who rarely, if ever, ate them.

One possible reason? Hot peppers contain lots of capsaicin, which has anti-inflammatory properties, along with healthy doses of beta carotene and quercetin.

Capsaicin protects the brain. Chinese researchers have found an association between people who eat a lot of capsaicin-rich chili peppers and lower rates of Alzheimer's. To understand why this might happen, they studied the effects of capsaicin on mice bred to have the early onset form of the disease. Sure enough, the mice who took the compound for six months were better able to learn and remember than the ones who didn't.

The scientist believe capsaicin works in two ways.

- It may reduce the production of beta-amyloid, the protein fragment that forms plaques in the brains of people with Alzheimer's.

- It may protect against brain inflammation and nerve damage.

Experts have long advised an overall healthy lifestyle to reduce the risk of cardiovascular disease and Alzheimer's. So add some chili peppers to guacamole, salsas, stir-fries, and curries. Now you're cooking!

Hot off the press: How fiery is that pepper?

With so many varieties of hot peppers to pick from, how do you decide which ones you want to flavor your foods?

Look for the Scoville heat unit (SHU) to learn how hot a pepper is before trying it. Numbers range from 0 for sweet bell peppers to over a million for the hottest of the hot — the Dragon's Breath, Carolina Reaper, and Death Spiral peppers.

To get started, this handy chart describes some of the most widely-enjoyed chili peppers. You can go to *scovillescale.org* for more information.

Pepper	SHU	Characteristics
Banana	0 to 500 (very mild)	This pepper has a tangy, slightly sweet taste. It is often pickled and sliced into rings to be used on salads, sandwiches, and pizza. Banana peppers can also be eaten raw as a snack.
Poblano	1,000 to 1,500 (mild)	One of the most popular peppers in Mexico, poblanos have an earthy taste. They are large with thick skins that hold up well for stuffing and roasting. When dried, this veggie is called "ancho."
Jalapeno	2,500 to 8,000 (medium)	Jalapenos are used in appetizers, soups, salads, and jellies. Their grassy flavor becomes richer when roasted. The smoked version of this pepper is dubbed "chipotle."
Serrano	10,000 to 23,000 (medium)	These peppers are similar in color and taste to the jalapeno, but with more bite. Serranos are often used in relishes, garnishes, sauces, and salsa. They're a good choice for people who are used to eating spicy food.
Cayenne	30,000 to 50,000 (medium-hot)	You know the hot, pungent red pepper flakes in glass jars at pizzerias? That's cayenne. The pepper is sold mostly as a dried, ground powder in the supermarket spice aisle. Ground cayenne is much spicier than chili powder, which can include garlic and cumin.
Habanero	100,000 to 350,000 (very hot)	Habaneros have a citrus-like flavor, as well as a flowery aroma. They complement sweet dishes like mango salsa. The pepper turns from green to orange or red as it ripens.

Peppers for your peepers — day or night, improve your sight

Keep an eye out for peppers on your next trip to the store and you could be doing your vision a huge favor. Peppers are not only rich in flavor and color, they're just loaded with eye-protecting nutrients.

Looking to cut salt from your diet? Spice it up! A brand-new study found that adults over age 60 had a hard time distinguishing between low-salt and high-salt sauces when a little chipotle seasoning was added. So bring on the chili peppers — your blood pressure will thank you.

Take your pick from sweet bell peppers to hot chili peppers and more. If it's a *Capsicum annum*, it's jam-packed with vitamins, minerals, and antioxidants that provide health benefits from head to toe.

Protect against cataracts with vitamin C. Cataracts are the leading cause of blindness around the world. In fact, more than half of all Americans will develop at least one cataract by age 80. But there's still plenty you can do to help protect your eyesight.

A British study of 1,000 pairs of twin sisters age 60 and above showed that those who got more vitamin C from their food had a 20% lower risk of developing this condition. When the researchers followed up with some of the same women 10 years later, those still eating a high vitamin C diet had a whopping 33% reduced risk of their cataracts getting worse.

The scientists believe this nutrient helps prevent oxidation, which can cause the lens in your eye to become cloudy. So eat more peppers. Half of a large sweet yellow pepper provides you with more than your recommended daily amount of vitamin C. It's nature's all-natural cataract preventer.

Reduce the risk of age-related macular degeneration with lutein and zeaxanthin. Pronounced loo-TEEN and zee-uh-ZAN-thin, these two nutrients — also found in peppers — are powerful antioxidants in their own right. They target the center of your retina, called the macula, and help clean up damage that comes from normal aging.

It's easy to add peppers into your daily meals, especially since a recent study published in the highly respected journal *Food Chemistry: X* found that sweet red peppers keep their high nutrient levels up to 21 days in the fridge. So eat up and help keep your vision sharp at any age.

 Boost the benefits

When it comes to preparing red peppers, experts agree — "wokking" is good for you. In fact, stir-frying is the best way to cook these veggies if you want to get the most vitamin C.

That's what Korean researchers found after roasting, steaming, boiling, and stir-frying red peppers. They discovered that boiling reduced vitamin C levels the most — as much as 67% after 15 minutes — while steaming was little better. Roasting came in second best, while stir-frying led to a mere 14% loss of this important antioxidant.

That's next to nothing when you consider that a single cup of raw sweet red pepper has more than twice the amount of vitamin C you need each day. Red chili peppers are also an excellent source of this nutrient.

So "wok" away from steamers and pots of boiling water in favor of stir-frying. Your immune system will thank you!

A closer look
Going organic

So what makes organic produce special? It's really pretty simple. Fruits and veggies that are "certified organic" are grown without the use of synthetic pesticides, fertilizers, or herbicides. Although this produce is no more nutritious than its conventionally produced twin, eating organic foods helps keep harmful chemicals out of your diet. Plus it's good for the environment.

But organic options are more expensive — sometimes 50% more. That's because all-natural farming is usually small scale and labor intensive. But you can minimize the costs at the supermarket. Just be selective in your purchases, says the Environmental Working Group.

Dubbed the "Dirty Dozen" by the nonprofit research group, these conventionally grown fruits and veggies have the highest concentrations of pesticide residue after being washed or peeled. So reserve your organic grocery budget for the following foods.

- strawberries
- nectarines
- pears
- bell and hot peppers
- spinach
- apples
- cherries
- celery
- tomatoes
- grapes
- peaches
- kale, collards, and mustard greens

In contrast, the Environmental Working Group says these types of produce carry the lowest pesticide punch. So if you're looking to save, the following would be the safest among the nonorganic crops.

- avocados
- onions
- asparagus
- cabbage
- mango
- sweet corn
- papaya
- kiwi
- mushrooms
- watermelon
- pineapple
- frozen sweet peas
- honeydew melon
- cantaloupe
- sweet potatoes

You can make regular produce safer by washing away pesticides for just a few pennies. Researchers found that rubbing fruits and veggies under running water for one minute does the job fine.

Potatoes

How sweet it is! Beta carotene ain't no small potatoes

Mashed, boiled, baked, or grilled — no matter how you enjoy sweet potatoes, one thing is for sure. These supercharged root vegetables are interesting fare.

For starters, a sweet potato isn't a potato at all. It's a member of the morning glory family, a species of flowering plants. This vegetable comes in some 6,500 varieties and a rainbow of colors, some with pink, purple, or yellow skins and others with white, gold, or orange flesh.

But don't let these far-out facts cloud the real reason you want to eat sweet potatoes. The Center for Science in the Public Interest says this veggie is one of the most nutritious foods you can eat. It's low in saturated fat and sodium, but rich in vitamin C, fiber, potassium, manganese, and vitamin B6.

Are sweet potato leaves edible? Sure are. When cooked, this nutritious green has a mild flavor much like spinach. Try stir-frying the leaves with sesame oil, ginger, and a dash of lemon juice. Or saute them in olive oil with onions, garlic, and red pepper flakes.

But let's not leave out the best part. Sweet potatoes are an absolutely fantastic source of beta carotene, one of a group of plant pigments called carotenoids that give many fruits and veggies their vibrant colors.

And what does your body do with all that beta carotene? It converts it into vitamin A. Hard to believe, but a medium-sized baked sweet potato weighing a little more than 5 ounces provides an incredible 1,370 micrograms (mcg) of vitamin A. That's well over the recommended daily amount of 700 mcg for senior women and 900 mcg for older men.

Here's why beta carotene and vitamin A are so spectacular.

- Research has found that eating a diet rich carotenoids — particularly beta carotene — is associated with lower visceral fat. That's the kind of fat that wraps around your internal organs and is a risk factor for cardiovascular disease.

- Vitamin A is vital for bone growth and strength. Scientists believe it may stimulate the growth of new bone cells. That's really important because too much bone loss can lead to osteoporosis, a condition marked by weak and brittle bones that fracture easily.

- Brain protective properties found in beta carotene may reduce the risk of neurodegenerative conditions, including Alzheimer's disease. What's more, a recent study found a link between this nutrient and lower rates of brain cell loss among seniors without dementia.

- Higher levels of carotenoids in the blood — including beta carotene — have been linked to a decreased risk of obesity and metabolic syndrome. What's metabolic syndrome? It's a dangerous condition marked by high blood sugar, abnormal cholesterol levels, elevated blood pressure, and excess fat around the waist.

Let's wrap up with another fun fact — February marks National Sweet Potato month. But you won't want to wait until then to serve this tasty veggie. It goes great in salads, stews, soups, casseroles, and desserts. So eat up!

Kitchen hacks

Cleaning potatoes is necessary to remove dirt, bacteria, and pesticides. Don't skip this step, even if you plan on peeling your spuds.

One of the best ways to remove unwanted debris from potatoes is to exfoliate them. Yes, the same method you use to achieve soft and clean skin removes the bad stuff from root vegetables, including potatoes.

Soak potatoes briefly in warm water before using an exfoliating glove to rub away the gunk.

This spud's for you — all hail the tasty tater's surprising benefits

When you think of foods rich in important nutrients, a white potato may not be on your list or your plate. But it should be. Believe it or not, this veggie has a lot to offer when prepared properly.

In fact, white potatoes are loaded with vital vitamins and minerals that keep you healthy and guard against disease. So feel free to include them as part of a wholesome diet.

This tasty tuber is full of vitamin C. An 8-ounce, medium-sized white potato — with the skin — contains 29 milligrams (mg) of vitamin C. That's almost 40% of the amount a senior woman should get every day, and nearly a third of the vitamin C older men need daily. This powerful antioxidant keeps your skin healthy and assists in iron absorption.

Potassium keeps your heart beating strong. This mineral is super important when it comes to healthy muscles, including your heart and those in your digestive system. That very same potato has nearly 900 mg of potassium — about double the amount contained in a medium-sized banana.

Get more B6 for carbohydrate and protein metabolism. White potatoes are a fantastic source of vitamin B6, with a single cup providing roughly a quarter of the daily needs of senior men and women. In addition to helping break down carbohydrates and protein, this mighty vitamin keeps your immune system robust.

Get the best from spuds by following some simple rules. Keep your portion sizes in check, and bake, roast, or boil your potatoes instead of frying. Be sure to eat the skins for extra fiber and nutrients, and garnish your taters with spices, herbs, and olive oil instead of butter.

Purple reigns, so go bold for smashing results

Just saw a purple potato in the produce aisle? No need to get your eyes checked. These visually stunning spuds, native to the Andes region of South America, are becoming more and more popular in the U.S.

And for good reason. For starters, they look impressive on the plate. Purple potatoes come in several varieties, and can have different shades of flesh — from solid magenta to violet marbling. But the power of this veggie isn't just cosmetic. They're really good for you, too.

Color brings potent benefits. It's the anthocyanins — the pigment that gives these potatoes, well, their "purpleness" — that make this veggie so healthy. These natural compounds also give blueberries, red cabbage, and blood oranges their vivid hues.

Anthocyanins work as powerful antioxidants that prevent or delay cell damage from unstable molecules. Dubbed free radicals, these molecules have been linked to several conditions, including cardiovascular disease, vision problems, inflammatory disorders, and diabetes.

So once in a while, swap out the potatoes you normally eat. The purple kind taste pretty much the same, but are smaller and less starchy than the russet and Idaho versions.

Pick the perfect tater and more. Use these tips to get the most out of this colorful food.

- Buy firm spuds that are smooth and sprout free. Or you can grow them by planting tubers in well-draining and slightly acidic soil.

- The best way to enjoy purple potatoes is to steam, bake, or boil them. They're great mashed, in salads, and paired with other veggies.

 Watch out

Let's face it. Potatoes have a lot of starch. But you probably knew that, along with the fact that this type of carb causes your blood sugar levels to rise quickly. And that increases your risk of weight gain, type 2 diabetes, and cardiovascular disease. What a bummer.

But wait. You can make potato starch work towards creating a healthier you. Just stick your spuds in the fridge after cooking. That's right — cooling them increases their levels of resistant starch. These carbs don't get digested, so they won't break down into sugar in your small intestine and then raise your blood glucose levels.

Next stop? The large intestine, where they ferment into a five-star dinner for the friendly gut bacteria that keep your digestive tract running smoothly.

Once you've chilled your cooked potatoes, serve them cold or reheated. Yes, you can have your potato and eat it too!

Tomatoes

3 surprising reasons to drink tomato juice

Enjoying tomato juice — made from fresh tomatoes with no added salt or sugar — is a fantastic way to reap the amazing health benefits of this garden favorite. You get the spectacular flavor of fresh tomatoes in a glass and benefit from its star lineup of nutrients and phytochemicals. Here are a few surprising reasons why a glass of tomato juice deserves a space at your table.

Tackle "bad" cholesterol with tasty tomato juice. Loaded with the powerful antioxidant lycopene, tomato juice is kind to your ticker. After following a low-tomato diet for three weeks, participants in one study drank about 1 1/2 cups of tomato juice and ate about 2 tablespoons of tomato ketchup every day for three weeks. Total cholesterol dropped about 6% and "bad" LDL cholesterol by about 13% with the high-tomato diet compared to the low.

A great start. The Centers for Disease Control and Prevention reports that a 10% decrease in total cholesterol can result in a staggering 30% reduction in the incidence of heart disease.

Sipping tomato juice boosts immune function. Foods that support your immune system may give you a protective advantage when cold and flu season rolls around. Tomatoes and tomato juice are both an excellent addition to your immune-boosting regimen. The vitamin A and iron in tomatoes encourage healthy immune cell function and promote your body's innate healing response. The potent antioxidants beta carotene and vitamins C and E protect cells from free radical damage, which can compromise your immune system.

Make tomato juice your go-to exercise recovery drink. A familiar feeling happens a day or so after a hard workout. Your muscles are sore, and you probably feel a little stiff, right? A tall drink of tomato juice could change everything.

So move over energy drinks. Tomato juice is in the house. A study conducted in Greece compared two groups of athletes — giving one group tomato juice and the other an energy drink during and after workouts for two months. The group that drank tomato juice had lower levels of markers that signal muscle damage.

So when should you pluck a tomato from the vine? If you wait until it turns red, you'll get the maximum amount of the antioxidant lycopene. On the other hand, you'll get more vitamin C if you harvest the tomato while it's green and let it ripen off the vine.

It works this way. When you exercise, your body produces unstable molecules that can harm your muscles. Antioxidants in tomato juice help your body remove them and speed up post-exercise recovery.

 Bright idea

The antioxidant lycopene that's behind many tomato benefits is also a pigment, which makes it a safer alternative to dangerous synthetic food colorings. In fact, researchers say that using byproducts of tomato processing to add vibrant color to food could be a healthy and sustainable opportunity.

Red tomatoes have already been used to color foods like pasta, crackers, hamburgers, breads, and cheeses. These products may list tomato concentrate or tomato lycopene color in the ingredients, so keep an eye out.

Boost the benefits

Tomatoes seem pretty simple on the surface — a vibrant and soft outer coating covers seeds and flesh. The truth is, this summertime favorite is more than meets the eye. Let's unpack some fascinating facts.

- The seeds are thought to contain anti-inflammatory properties, so be sure to enjoy them with the rest of the fruit — or vegetable, if you prefer to classify it by its culinary use.

- Eating tomatoes can help you achieve your daily water quota. They're more than 90% water.

- Avoid the refrigerator for tastier tomatoes. Storing them there reduces the nutrient value, slows ripening, and diminishes the taste. Choose a cool and shady location with a temperature between 65 to 70 degrees for your fruit to ripen.

- The inner cavities of tomatoes, known as the locules, contain more vitamin C than the outer or pericarp tissue.

Garden darling takes cancer head-on and wins

With over 10,000 varieties grown worldwide, tomatoes have earned a prized spot in the home garden. Although they are revered for their taste and culinary flexibility, this fruit may also hold the key to fighting one of the deadliest diseases of all time — cancer.

Out of all the nonstarchy vegetables, Americans eat tomatoes and tomato products the most. And since research continues to uncover evidence that this favorite summer vegetable may help prevent eight kinds of cancer, this fondness for tomatoes is a good thing. The cancer-protecting prowess comes mainly from the superpower antioxidant lycopene, which gives tomatoes their beautiful red hue.

Tomato lovers have a reduced risk of prostate cancer.
Although prostate cancer is the most frequently diagnosed cancer in men, it has an almost 100% survival rate when caught early. Adding tomatoes to your diet might even reduce the risk of developing this cancer. One study found that men who ate more than 10 servings of tomatoes and tomato products weekly had an 18% lower risk.

Just a single cup of tomato juice a day offers breast cancer protection. To see how tomatoes might stack up to this condition, researchers recruited a group of postmenopausal women at a high risk for breast cancer. After 10 weeks of eating about 25 milligrams of lycopene daily — the amount found in a cup of tomato juice — the women had increased levels of the cancer-protecting protein adiponectin in their blood.

Four tomatoes daily lower kidney cancer risk. Women who ate the highest amounts of lycopene-rich foods such as tomatoes had a 45% lower risk of developing kidney cancer than those who ate the least, according to research. Study leaders say the amount the ladies ate is on par with snacking on about four tomatoes a day.

Eat your sunscreen and ward off skin cancer. A team of scientists have discovered that eating 5 tablespoons of tomato paste daily may protect against damaging UV rays. When participants ate the tomato paste daily for three months, they had a 33% greater protection against sunburn. A big deal since this damage can lead to skin cancer.

Slice your risk of lung cancer. You can breathe a sigh of relief after hearing this news. Research shows that eating tomatoes is linked to a lower

A large, decade-long study has found that the natural decline in lung function that occurs with age is slower among people who eat a lot of tomatoes. The results were particularly striking among former smokers. So eat more tomatoes — their antioxidants may just help you breathe easy.

risk of lung cancer. Test tube studies reveal that the lycopene may deter the growth of the cancer cells.

Homegrown gardens are ripe for liver cancer defense.
Lycopene may be the star of the show, but don't discount the power of tomatoes over supplements. An animal study suggests that tomato powder can reduce liver cancer development. Researchers point out that the tomato powder was more effective than lycopene supplementation. They think other tomato nutrients like vitamin E, vitamin C, beta carotene, minerals, and dietary fibers may also be at work.

Colon and stomach cancers waylaid by yummy veggie.
Eating tomatoes is linked to a lower risk of stomach and colon cancer. There you have it. Tomatoes — the brightest way to make your taste buds and tummy happy.

Tomatoes might just be the new fountain of youth

Could eating one common vegetable be your ticket to preventing wrinkles, avoiding sunburn, and stopping skin cancer before it starts? Research says yes to tomatoes. As you know, eating this tasty food protects your skin from damaging UV rays, which can cause sunburn and skin cancer. But here's something else to think about — those harmful rays may also lead to premature skin aging.

Exposure to UV rays may be responsible for up to 80% of the visible signs of aging, including wrinkles, pigmentation issues, and dryness. Protecting your skin on the outside with a sunscreen that has an SPF of at least 30 is a must. But since tomatoes act as a natural sunscreen, shielding against sunburn and its ensuing damage, you might want to make tomato-based pasta sauce, sun-dried tomatoes, and hearty tomato soup part of your repertoire, too.

UV protection is just a part of the equation, though. These veggies are packed with vitamin C — 19% to 23% of your daily needs in a whole tomato. Not only does vitamin C act as a skin-shielding antioxidant, but it also plays an important role in the production of collagen, a protein that helps keep your skin plump and youthful. Researchers confirm that tomatoes appear to boost procollagen, a precursor to collagen. They say that increasing levels of this peptide could help push back your skin's aging process.

So if you want beautiful and radiant skin, bring on the tomatoes and don't forget the sunscreen.

Heirloom seeds:
How to save for tasty veggies every year

Mm. Juicy, vibrant heirloom tomatoes. These naturally pollinated, nonhybrid varieties come from saved seeds that have been passed down for generations. Generally, that means incredible taste and more nutrients than you'll find in your local grocery store options.

And it means you can save the seeds yourself for more mouthwatering tomatoes next season. Follow these easy steps to collect and preserve seeds.

- Scoop out the gelatinous tomato pulp containing the seeds into a glass container.

- Add a cup of water to the container and cover it.

- Store the container in a location away from direct sunlight for four days.

- Strain seeds from the water using a sieve and rinse.

- Place seeds on a paper plate to dry. Break up any seed clumps.

- Store dry seeds in a zipper bag in a cool and dark spot. Be sure to label them.

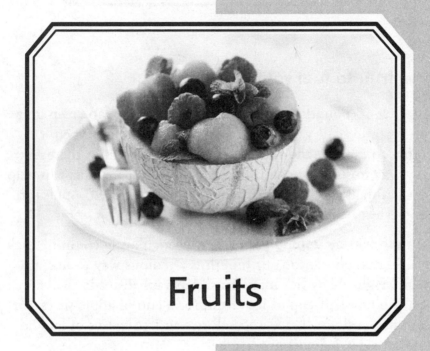

Fruits

Apples

The fruit to fuel your weight loss

Another 10 pounds? That number on the scale can creep up as the years go by if you're not making smart choices when it comes to exercise and the food you eat. Thankfully, there's an easy way to slim your waistline. Swapping fat for fiber can help you naturally cut calories and feel full and satisfied. Apples are the perfect fruit to do just that.

Scale down by upping your fiber. Meticulously counting each morsel that goes into your mouth is a tedious way to manage your weight. Why not make sensible swaps instead? Switch your nightly half-cup of ice cream for a cup of apple slices, for example, and you'll save 155 calories and 16 grams of fat and gain an extra 3 grams of fiber.

You'll be glad you did. And fiber may be the main reason. In one study, researchers examined whether different types of diets would result in higher weight loss among overweight and obese participants. They found that eating lots of fiber was the greatest predictor of weight loss, regardless of the percentage of protein, carbs, or fat the participants ate. As an extra benefit, those who ate more fiber also stuck to their diets better.

If you have trouble getting enough fiber, apples are an 5 way to meet your goals. One medium apple has 21% of the daily recommended amount if you're a woman over 50 and 15% for a man of the same age.

Trade your potato chip habit with baked apple chips for a fiber-filled snack. And ditch those low-fiber pretzels and cookies for apple slices dipped in low-fat yogurt or roasted apples with cinnamon.

The trick to feeling fuller longer. Your weight management plan won't work if you're always hungry. And how you eat your apples matters more than you might think.

Researchers found that it took people longer to digest apples in their whole form compared to puree or juice with the same amount of calories. The small group of participants in the study also reported feeling fuller and more satisfied after eating the whole apple.

No surprise really. Slower digestion time makes you feel fuller longer. Plus chewing whole apples takes more effort and time than taking a swig of apple juice. That — along with the complex texture of the apples — increases satisfaction, say researchers.

Discover the power of the peel for joint pain

Rain must be on its way. After all, legend has it that stiff and painful joints never lie. While predicting the weather might sound like a perk, achy joints can really put a damper on moving through your day. Instead of waiting around for drier weather, try grabbing an apple for the relief you need.

In one study, 12 people who suffered from stiff and painful joints had better range of motion and pain levels after eating dried apple peel powder daily for 12 weeks, with some improvements in range of motion after only two weeks. The amount participants took in the study was equal to three apple peels each day.

How do peels perk up your aching joints? Scientists believe the improvements are related to an increase in antioxidant activity and reduced inflammation in the body.

Heart guard: Medicine from the orchard, not the pharmacy

The average American eats over 16 pounds of apples a year. And no wonder. They help ease arthritis, boost lung power, and aid digestion. Bet you can't guess what else this tasty super fruit can do — protect your heart.

Squash heart disease by following this common proverb. An apple a day to keep the doctor away may sound like an old wives tale, but there may actually be some truth to it. In fact, munching on an apple daily could work as well as statins at preventing heart attacks and strokes, according to British researchers.

Using existing population data, they estimated that by eating one apple every day, people age 50 and older could avoid or delay 8,500 heart attacks and strokes each year. One reason apples are so great for blood flow may be because they tackle high cholesterol.

In one study, 45 postmenopausal women ate dried apples — equivalent to two medium-sized apples or a dozen dried apple rings — each day and lowered bad LDL cholesterol by 24% within six months. After one year, good HDL cholesterol increased by 3% and a kind of fat called triglycerides decreased by 9%. Researchers suspect that apples' cholesterol-lowering superpowers come from pectin, a type of soluble fiber that helps your body get rid of cholesterol instead of absorbing it into the bloodstream.

Of course that doesn't mean you should skip your statins. Always consult with your doctor and take medications as prescribed. But if you're looking for ways to improve your heart health, make sure apples are on the grocery list.

Buy them by the bushel to stave off diabetes. Eating apples could also help you ward off high blood sugar. Researchers analyzed three landmark nutrition studies that followed more than 180,000 adults over a collective 64 years and found that eating lots of apples reduced the chances of developing diabetes.

That's amazing news since high blood sugar can damage blood vessels, which is why people with diabetes are two to four times more likely to develop heart disease.

How might apples put the kibosh on diabetes? Researchers say the relationship could have something to do with anthocyanins, a type of antioxidant found in apples and other fruits like pears and blueberries. Animal studies have found that anthocyanins lower blood glucose and increase insulin sensitivity.

 Kitchen hacks

Red, yellow, pink, green. There are almost as many colors and varieties of apples as there are ways to eat them. Use this guide to choose the best apple for your next pie, sauce, or afternoon snack.

- **Braeburn:** Hard and tart. You'll want these for your next apple cobbler.

- **Gala:** Sweet and crisp. The perfect snacking apple.

- **Granny Smith:** Tart and firm. You'll love these for homemade applesauce.

- **Honeycrisp:** Sweet, crisp, and slightly tart. A great everyday snacking apple.

- **Jazz:** Crunchy and juicy. Try them baked in pies.

- **Jonathan:** Slightly tart. Goes great in sauces and is good for baking and snacking.

- **McIntosh:** Crispy, juicy, and firm. Tasty for snacking and making pies, sauce, or juice.

- **Red Delicious:** Sweet and tart. Slice and toss in salads.

Sweet solutions for all that ails you

You'll want to buy your apples by the dozen after learning about the disease-fighting power this little fruit has. The benefits of an apple-snacking habit range from your heart to your kidneys to your bones and beyond. When it comes to keeping your vision and mind sharp, the antioxidants in apples are ready for action.

Powerful nutrients to support your eyes. Dry eyes are more than just an annoying inconvenience. If left untreated, reduced tear production could lead to irritation, scarring, and impaired vision. Interestingly, researchers found that quercetin, an antioxidant found in the peel of apples, improved tear production and corneal smoothness when applied as eye drops in an animal study.

Not to mention, one medium-sized apple contains 9% to 11% of your daily recommended amount of vitamin C. The American Optometric Association has praised this antioxidant for its role in protecting against cataracts.

Juice up for brain health. While some forgetfulness is considered a normal part of life, munching on apples might just give your brain a little boost.

To test it out, researchers gave mice diluted apple juice daily for one month. And even though some of the mice were bred to develop Alzheimer's-like symptoms, researchers still noted an improvement in cognitive performance. The amount of juice was equivalent to drinking 16 ounces of juice or eating two to three apples each day.

Scientists believe the protection provided by apple juice is twofold. Antioxidants reduce damage from free radicals in the brain. Furthermore, apple juice may slow down the decline of the neurotransmitter acetylcholine. Your noggin needs this chemical to communicate between nerve cells, and decreased levels are linked to Alzheimer's disease.

Apricots

The magic fruit to help you feel and look your best

The English settlers must have known the value of apricots when they went through the trouble of bringing them to the New World back in the 17th century. Nowadays, scientists can confirm that they were worth all that effort. With loads of nutrients and only 16 calories per apricot, these tiny fruits pack a wholesome punch that will leave you glowing from the inside out.

Get plenty of iron to fight fatigue. Sluggishness could come from a lack of iron. This essential mineral is an important component of hemoglobin, a protein that carries oxygen throughout your body so that your tissues and muscles can use it to create energy.

A cup of fresh apricot halves will get you about 8% of the iron you need each day. But dried apricots are even better. Half a cup has 22% of your daily iron.

Improve your skin, hair, and nails with vitamin C. A cup of fresh apricots has 17% to 21% of your daily value of vitamin C. This nutrient helps your body absorb iron, which is important for healthy hair and nails. And that's not the only reason it may be the key to a glowing appearance.

Researchers found that eating more vitamin C is linked to better skin aging, including fewer wrinkles and less dryness. Vitamin C's antioxidant powers as well as its role in collagen creation and cell regeneration are what helps keep your skin smooth and supple.

Help your heart by focusing on fiber. You don't have to suck down a serving of gritty Wheaties to get your fill of fiber. Dried apricots have just as much. At 4.75 grams per 1/2 cup, this sweet snack will get you 16% to 23% of the fiber you need each day.

And while fiber has a reputation for helping you stay regular, it does more than just keep digestion moving smoothly. The fiber in apricots may lower blood pressure and combat high cholesterol.

- Researchers at Tulane University reviewed 25 clinical studies on fiber and high blood pressure. They found that people who increased their fiber intake for at least eight weeks had reductions in blood pressure.

- Besides high blood pressure, high LDL cholesterol also increases your risk for heart disease. The soluble fiber in apricots can crush LDL cholesterol by helping your body get rid of it before it enters your bloodstream where it can clog your arteries.

Kitchen hacks

Fresh apricots are at their peak from June to mid-August. Here's how to pick and store them.

Buying. Look for a fruit that's yellow to orange, with no green. A ripe apricot should yield only slightly when you press it gently, and it should smell sweet.

Storing. You can place unripe fruit on the counter in a paper bag to ripen more quickly. Once ripe, store for up to a week in the refrigerator.

Freezing. If you're blessed with more apricots than you can eat, freezing is a great way to store them. Slice them in half to remove the pit. Then dip them in an ascorbic acid solution — or lemon juice if that's all you have on hand — to help preserve their beautiful color. Freeze them in an airtight bag for up to three months.

Protect your peepers with 3 essential vitamins

Bird-watching, reading, or taking your dog for a walk — no matter what your favorite activity is, you count on your eyes to help you do it. Start snacking on sweet, juicy apricots to keep your eyes healthy and vision sharp so you can do more of what you love for years to come. With a trifecta of vitamins for optimal eye health, you'll be seeing this stone fruit in a new light.

Vitamin A. Beta carotene is one of the many carotenoids that give apricots their bright yellow-orange color. Amazingly, your body converts it into vitamin A, and that's when the real magic happens.

Vitamin A helps your eyes see in dark or low-light situations, which comes in handy when you're driving at dusk or playing card games by lamplight. Every cup of fresh apricots provides 17% of the vitamin A recommended daily for men over the age of 50 and 21% for women of the same age.

Vitamins A and E are fat soluble. That means your body will absorb them better if you eat them with fat. Simple enough. Make your own trail mix with dried apricots. Be sure to include healthy fats in the form of pecans, walnuts, almonds, or sunflower seeds.

Vitamin C. An antioxidant powerhouse, vitamin C can help you see more clearly through its free radical-busting activity. That means it may help neutralize oxidation before the damage can lead to cataracts or the progression of age-related macular degeneration.

One cup of fresh apricots has 15.5 milligrams (mg) of vitamin C. That's a great head start in reaching the recommended 75 mg for women and 90 mg for men.

Vitamin E. As another antioxidant, vitamin E may also be helpful in protecting against damage that causes cataracts and macular degeneration. You'll get 19% of your daily value of vitamin E in just 1/2 cup of dried apricot halves.

Fierce flavonols: Nutrients that fight inflammation

Your immune system keeps you in fine feather when it sends inflammatory cells to attack bacteria and heal damaged tissue. But what happens when this lifesaving response continues long after the danger has passed? Chronic inflammation.

It's a dangerous condition that has been linked to problems like heart disease, Parkinson's disease, diabetes, memory loss, and some cancers. Thankfully, apricots have plenty of flavonols, nutrients that act as antioxidants to help combat inflammation.

To see if flavonols are all they're cracked up to be, researchers analyzed the diets of more than 2,000 men and women from data collected over the course of three years. Then they used information on the participants' inflammatory blood markers to give them inflammation scores.

Eating more flavonol-rich foods was related to lower overall inflammation scores. Getting high amounts of flavonols was also linked to lower markers of oxidative stress, an imbalance between free radicals and antioxidants.

So go ahead and fill up on tasty apricots, along with some other high-flavonol foods like apples and pears. Simmer the trio in honey and spices to make a compote that tastes delicious on yogurt. Or try them mixed into a fruit salad.

Avocados

Miffed at your midriff? Banish belly fat with this buttery fruit

Apple or pear? No, it's not a question about your favorite fruit. It's all about your body and the changes that often occur in your 40s and 50s — when the fat from your hips and thighs appears to resettle around your belly. Next thing you know, you're shaped more like an apple than a pear.

It's a problem generally associated with women and tied to the hormonal changes that come with menopause. But men can get this stubborn paunch, too. And it can be downright dangerous.

That's because belly fat isn't limited to a layer of jiggly padding under the skin. It includes visceral fat — the kind that wraps around your internal organs and is linked to heart disease, high blood pressure, and type 2 diabetes. Yikes!

But here's the good news. Eating avocados may just make that deep belly fat go away. That's what researchers discovered after splitting more than 100 overweight or obese adults into two groups. One ate a meal with a Hass avocado each day for 12 weeks while the other had a nearly identical meal without the green fruit.

At the end of the study, the scientists found that the women who ate an avocado each day experienced a reduction in visceral fat.

So what makes this creamy fruit a weight-loss superfood? It could be related to the 10 grams of fiber — that's nearly 50%

of the recommended daily allowance for a woman over the age of 50 — found in an average-sized Hass avocado.

And a lot of that fiber is insoluble. That's the kind of roughage that doesn't break down. It helps food move more quickly through your digestive system, which may decrease the amount of calories your body absorbs.

In addition, avocados are high in healthy monounsaturated fats that scientists believe may redistribute abdominal fat away from the visceral kind.

Oddly enough, the men in the study who ate a daily avocado didn't have the same results as the women. The researchers aren't exactly sure why. But they hope to conduct further studies that look at markers of gut health and the effects of avocados on the metabolism. That, they say, would help them determine if different results remain between the two sexes.

Tap into avocado for surprising health benefits

Lots of people think of avocados as vegetables. After all, they're not sweet like bananas or sour like lemons. But don't be fooled by this food's earthy, slightly nutty flavor.

The avocado is most definitely a fruit — in fact it's a giant berry with a single seed. But more importantly, this tasty treat can help reduce both your appetite and your risk of heart disease.

Feel full and satisfied. Hungry again? If you're reaching for a snack before you've even cleaned the plates from your kitchen table, you may want to add avocado to your menu.

Researchers put this delicious fruit to the test with 26 healthy but overweight adults. They found that simply adding half an avocado to the participants' lunches significantly reduced their desire to eat for a whopping five hours.

The scientists say the healthy fats and fiber in the avocado may have left the participants feeling fuller. And while the avocado added around 100 calories to their lunches, the people in the study offset that gain with fewer calories later in the day. Feeling more satisfied after eating can help you snack less and make weight management easier.

Keep arteries clear. Eating avocados could give you the advantage you need to keep your ticker in tiptop shape. That's according to Penn State researchers who discovered that people experienced a drop in their LDL cholesterol levels after eating a daily avocado over five weeks.

> The Hass is the king of California's avocado crop. It's also the most popular type of avocado sold in the United States. To open the fruit, make a single slice length-wise around the seed. Gently twist apart the two sides and remove the pit with a spoon. Holy guacamole, that's easy!

Specifically, the study found that avocados helped reduce LDL particles that had been oxidized. Similar to the way oxygen can damage food — like a cut apple turning brown — the researchers say oxidation can lead to plaque buildup that clogs the arteries.

"Oxidation is not good, so if you can help protect the body through the foods that you eat, that could be very beneficial," says Penny Kris-Etherton, distinguished professor of nutrition and co-author of the study.

Scientists also found that avocados are effective at controlling dangerous inflammation. They split overweight adults into two groups and put them both on a low-calorie meal plan. The difference? One set of people ate a daily avocado while the other skipped the fruit.

After three months, both groups lost similar amounts of weight. But the folks who ate the avocado also saw a drop in their levels of C-reactive protein — a blood test marker for inflammation that is associated with heart disease. The researchers say the results may be due to the healthy fatty acids in avocados.

 Bright idea

If the only way you're eating avocado is in guacamole, you're missing out. This fruit is a natural, one-ingredient swap when it comes to cooking and baking, plus it's good for your ticker. Try these unconventional ways to trade out harmful saturated fats for heart-healthy avocados.

- Instead of butter, smear blended avocado on your toast. You can also use this fruit as a substitute for shortening in baked goods. The beneficial fat in the avocado will add moisture and richness to your cakes, brownies, and muffins.

- Toss out your mayonnaise and use avocado as a nutritious binder for your egg, tuna, and chicken salads.

- Avocado can take the place of a dollop of sour cream in your soup or a slice of cheese in your sandwich. The creaminess and contrast to other ingredients makes it a perfect substitute.

- Instead of milk, blend avocado into your smoothie for a perfectly luscious texture.

Trust your gut with fabulous fiber

You may have heard that you've got trillions and trillions of microorganisms in your intestinal tract. No doubt, they live there for a reason. These "good" bacteria do everything from helping you digest food to regulating your immune system. Not only that, they keep colonies of "bad" bacteria — the kind that promote diseases — in check.

Now here's the really interesting part. You can keep these beneficial microbes in tiptop shape by eating avocado.

That's according to researchers who found that folks who ate the creamy fruit with one meal a day experienced an increase in the bacteria that break down soluble fiber — the kind that absorbs water. That's super important because when these microbes digest the roughage in plant-based foods, they produce short chain fatty acids that prevent bad bacteria from growing in your intestines. Those fatty acids also increase your ability to absorb minerals, reduce your appetite, and even combat inflammation.

"We can't break down dietary fibers, but certain gut microbes can," says Hannah Holscher, senior author of the 12-week study published in *The Journal of Nutrition*. "When we consume dietary fiber, it's a win-win for gut microbes and for us."

Half a cup of pureed Hass avocado has nearly 8 grams of fiber — enough to help ensure those good bacteria are well fed and producing fatty acids. This fruit also goes a long way toward meeting the recommended daily amount of 21 grams of fiber for women over age 50 and 30 grams for men of the same age.

The 'eyes' have it — protect your vision with this super fruit

It's hard to beat a colorful salad when it comes to getting important vitamins, minerals, and fiber. But here's a little-known secret. If you want to push those health benefits a step further, toss in some avocado. The fruit actually boosts the nutrition of the other ingredients.

How is that possible? Well, researchers at Purdue University discovered that adults who topped their salads with monounsaturated fats — which avocados are loaded with — were best able to absorb the antioxidants lutein and zeaxanthin. That's because these eye-healthy nutrients are fat soluble, meaning they break down a lot more efficiently when monounsaturated fats are present to help them along.

And here's why you'll want to load up on lutein and zeaxanthin. Both these compounds accumulate in your eye, where studies show they can protect your sight from the harmful effects of macular degeneration and cataracts. How? By fighting oxidative stress and inflammation.

So next time you make a salad, load it up with lutein- and zeaxanthin-rich ingredients like tomatoes, romaine lettuce, spinach, carrots, and orange peppers. Then slice some avocado on top. Doing so will give you the most nutritional bang for your buck, as well as provide a creamy counterpart to the crunchiness of the raw veggies. Your eyes — not to mention your taste buds — will thank you.

 Kitchen hacks

They say timing is everything. That certainly applies to avocados, where the window between having a rock hard fruit and a mushy one appears to be about an hour. But if you follow these tips, you'll enjoy a ripe fruit every time.

First, apply gentle pressure to the avocado's stem. If it's difficult to remove, the fruit is unripe. But your avocado is ready to eat if the stem flicks off easily to reveal a green color. If the flesh underneath the stem is brown, the fruit is overripe.

While the texture of the peel won't tell you how ripe the fruit is, you'll want to avoid avocados that are too soft or have dark blemishes on the skin. Both are signs that the fruit has seen better days.

Bananas

The time is ripe: Tap into these key nutrients now

Trying to stick to a healthy diet when you're in the mood for something sweet is enough to make anyone go bananas. But don't despair — this fruit may just be the world's most perfect snack.

Clocking in at around 100 calories, bananas are loaded with potassium for nerve and muscle health. And the golden fruit's health benefits don't stop there — bananas contain the following nutrients essential for keeping your body in top-notch condition.

Vitamin B6. Want to keep your brain healthy? Then make sure you get enough vitamin B6. It helps create neurotransmitters — chemical messengers in your brain — that help regulate your mood and emotions. Not only that, this vitamin is necessary for a functioning immune system and the production of red blood cells that carry oxygen.

And that's where bananas come in. Just one banana supplies seniors with roughly 25% of their recommended daily amount of B6. So blend them into smoothies, slice them on your morning cereal, and add them to fruit salads. Your body and mind will thank you!

Magnesium. With age comes wisdom, but it is often accompanied by dwindling magnesium levels. That's because the intestines of older folks tend to absorb less of this mineral, and their kidneys may excrete more of it in their urine. This deficiency can lead to a loss of bone density and an increased risk of fractures.

And your body relies on magnesium to regulate blood sugar levels and blood pressure. It's also important to getting a good night's sleep.

In fact, a two-month study of seniors with insomnia found that those who supplemented their daily diets with 500 milligrams of magnesium needed less time to fall asleep. They also experienced significant increases in the amount of time they spent snoozing.

While one banana won't cure insomnia, it provides adults over 30 with 8% to 10% of the magnesium they need daily. Eating this fruit alongside other magnesium-rich foods — think pumpkin seed kernels, almonds, spinach, cashews, and peanuts — can help you get even more of this precious mineral.

Fiber. You already know that roughage is important for good digestion and can be helpful when it comes to weight management. Research also shows that fiber can reduce your risk of diabetes and helps fight off breast cancer and heart disease.

So how much is enough? Women over the age of 50 should get 21 grams of fiber a day. Men of the same age should shoot for 30 grams. Sadly, most Americans fall far short of these goals. So load up on bananas. With around 3 grams of fiber, this sweet fruit will help you meet your target amount.

Enjoy these super 'a-peeling' workout benefits

Whether you hike in the woods or power-walk through the neighborhood, you'll want to take a banana along for the trip. This simple yellow fruit is the perfect snack to fuel your next workout.

That's what researchers who studied trained cyclists concluded. The scientists found that feeding the athletes bananas, along with water, worked just as well at fueling their performance as sugary sports drinks. That's great news if you're the active type, since bananas cost only pennies and are already wrapped in a travel-ready package.

"We found that not only was performance the same whether bananas or sports drinks were consumed, there were several advantages to consuming bananas," says David Nieman, Ph.D., director of the human performance lab where the study was held.

The bananas provided the cyclists with antioxidants — compounds that protect against cell damage — not found in the sports drinks. They also contained a greater nutritional boost and a healthier blend of sugars.

 Watch out

Do medical gloves and party balloons send you running in the opposite direction? The rubber latex in these products is harmless to most. But if you're allergic, coming into contact with them may cause you to suffer from hives, a runny nose, and shortness of breath.

Here's something few people know. Some vegetables and fruits, including bananas, contain proteins similar to those found in the sap of rubber trees. And eating them can sometimes cause an allergic reaction in people who are sensitive to latex.

The following are considered latex-reactive fare.

- fruits including apples, avocados, bananas, chestnuts, kiwi, melons, and papaya
- vegetables like carrots, celery, potatoes, and tomatoes

You're best bet? If you have an allergy to latex, ask your doctor about the safety of eating these foods.

This golden fruit cuts cancer risk

You've probably heard that you should eat at least five servings of fruit and veggies a day. But when it comes to kidney cancer, the types of plant-based foods you tuck away could be just as important as the number.

That's according to Swedish researchers who followed 61,000 women over more than a decade to see how their diets affected their risk of developing kidney cancer. They found that women who ate lots of fruits and veggies had a lower risk of getting the disease, although the results weren't considered significant in statistical terms.

But, within the group of fruits studied, the researchers discovered that bananas were especially effective at fending off the disease. In fact, women who noshed on four or more bananas per week were roughly half as likely to get kidney cancer as those who barely ate this fruit at all.

Think of bananas as the fruit that lowers blood pressure just like pills. After all, research suggests that foods high in potassium can help lower blood pressure. Bananas are particularly high in this essential mineral, as are cantaloupe, spinach, and sweet potato.

Scientists believe bananas' cancer-fighting power may come from their high levels of phenolic compounds with antioxidant properties.

Kitchen hacks

Stop! Before you toss that banana peel in the trash, take a minute to learn about these home remedies to treat your itchy, dry skin.

Say good-bye to bug bites. The only thing more annoying than a mosquito buzzing around your ear is the itchy bite it leaves behind. Try rubbing a banana peel, flesh side down, on the bite and let the natural oils go to work until the prickliness disappears.

Squash psoriasis symptoms. If you suffer from the autoimmune skin disease psoriasis, you're familiar with the raised, scaly patches that itch and burn. Turns out, applying the inside of the peel to your skin may provide much needed moisture and have an anti-inflammatory effect. Check with your doctor before trying.

Berries

Good food for life — eat to beat sickness

Berries sure bring a lot of health benefits to the table. In fact, berries are one of nature's best sources of antioxidants. These compounds, which fight off cell damage caused by unstable molecules, can reduce your odds of getting ill. So snack on these fruits daily to keep your body in fighting form.

Combat cancer. Scientists have found that black raspberries may slow the growth of colorectal cancer, the third most common type of cancer among men and women in the United States. A small nine-week study found that people with colorectal cancer who drank a daily mix of water and freeze-dried black raspberry powder experienced a decrease in tumor cell multiplication and an increase in tumor cell death.

While the exact cause for this improvement isn't 100% clear, researchers believe it may stem from the high amount of polyphenols, plant nutrients loaded with antioxidants, in black raspberries and the effect their metabolism has on cancer cells.

Decrease diabetes risk. Here's a reason to add fresh berries to your yogurt. A 19-year Finnish study of over 2,300 men found that those who included more berries in their diets were significantly less likely to develop type 2 diabetes. And believe it or not, the men who saw those health benefits ate, on average, just an ounce and a half of berries a day.

So why did berries help? The researchers believe the polyphenols in the fruit may improve the way sugar is metabolized. The compounds can also reduce oxidative stress and inflammation, two conditions that are thought to predispose folks to type 2 diabetes. Blueberries, blackberries, and strawberries are all major sources of polyphenols.

Boost heart health. To keep your ticker on a steady beat, bust out the blueberries. Researchers found that overweight adults who added a cup of this fruit to their diets each day over six months experienced improvements in blood vessel function, arterial stiffness, and HDL cholesterol. That reduced their risk of cardiovascular disease — a leading cause of heart disease and stroke — by up to 15%.

The people in the study had metabolic syndrome, a condition marked by high sugar and cholesterol levels and excess body fat around the waist. Scientists believe the antioxidants in blueberries deserve the credit for the fruit's healing powers.

The sweet truth about nature's candy

It's no surprise that eating too much sugar is bad for you. So, what about sweet fruit like berries?

Of course berries have natural sugar, but it's not nearly as bad for you as refined sugar. Berries are also among the top sources of vitamins and minerals. They're much lower in calories and more filling than, say, a candy bar or bottle of pop — both of which contain lots of processed sugar.

Berries also have lots of fiber to slow digestion, which helps control spikes in blood sugar. It's one of the reasons this juicy fruit has a low glycemic index — a scale that ranks carbohydrate-containing foods by how much they raise a person's blood sugar.

Now to decide which to snack on first. Strawberries, blueberries, raspberries, blackberries ... how will you pick?

Protect your brain from diseases of aging

People are living longer than ever. In fact, the average life expectancy in the United States is roughly 80 years. But with this increase in longevity comes extra challenges. Fortunately, though, berries are just what the doctor ordered for staving off the following illnesses.

Alzheimer's disease. Some 6 million Americans are living with Alzheimer's disease, a devastating brain disorder that destroys memory, thinking skills, and eventually the ability to carry out simple tasks. But the foods you eat may help cut your risk of developing this illness.

Researchers followed 2,800 adults for almost two decades to see whether the foods they ate impacted their risk of developing Alzheimer's disease. The scientists found that people were four times more likely to develop Alzheimer's and related forms of dementia if their diets lacked anthocyanins — a plant compound in berries that has antioxidant powers.

So load up on anthocyanin-rich strawberries or blueberries. Just 7 1/2 cups per month had a protective effect on the seniors in the study.

Parkinson's disease. Tremors, loss of balance, and slurred speech are a reality for people living with Parkinson's disease, a disorder of the nervous system that mainly affects older folks.

And here's how berries may help. Scientists analyzed the diets of more than 1,200 men and women and found that those who got the most anthocyanins from foods like berries had a lower risk of getting Parkinson's. The researchers believe these compounds protect the brain by increasing the release of dopamine, a neurotransmitter that is low in people with Parkinson's. Animal studies have also found that anthocyanins suppress nerve inflammation and oxidative stress.

But berries don't just cut your risk of getting Parkinson's. A separate study found that people with the disease who ate three or more servings of berries a week had a significantly greater survival rate than those who ate less than one serving a month.

This fruit is 'berry' good at keeping your mind sharp

Ever hear the expression "Happiness is good health and a bad memory?" It may hold water if you're looking to forget unfortunate events. But if you'd like to have both good health and a strong memory, start stocking your fridge with sweet and colorful berries.

Turns out they can keep your brain from aging. Scientists discovered this after keeping tabs on the diets of more than 16,000 women over the age of 70. When they tested the participants' brain skills over several years, the researchers found that the women who ate higher amounts of blueberries and strawberries developed memory problems less quickly. In fact, eating these fruits appeared to delay their cognitive aging by up to two and a half years.

The women didn't even have to eat mounds of berries every day to boost their memory and brain function. Just 1/2 cup of blueberries or two half-cup servings of strawberries every week was enough to get results. So eat up!

All kinds of berries are delicious and healthy. In fact, they help prevent Alzheimer's disease, infections, fatigue, belly fat, diabetes, heart disease, and even wrinkles. So try to eat berries every day — either added to breakfast oats, atop a lunchtime salad, or in a dinnertime salsa on grilled salmon.

Experts believe that stress and inflammation contribute to cognitive difficulties. So it makes sense, they say, that compounds in berries — specifically flavonoids with high antioxidant and anti-inflammatory properties — can protect the brain from harm.

Go, go goji! 2 super reasons to snack on this fruit

Thank goodness! Goji berries, which have been used in Chinese medicine for thousands of years, are finally on Western shelves. And not a moment too soon — these tiny fruits are packed with immune-boosting and vision-saving powers.

Stave off sickness. Cold and flu season isn't the only time to eat for immune health. Your cells and organs work year-round to protect you from dangerous germs that can cause infection, illness, and even death.

Enter goji berries. Just a single 1-ounce serving — about 5 tablespoons — of dried goji berries has more than 100% of the vitamin A you need daily. This vitamin maintains the mucosal cells in your eyes, lungs, and gut that provide a barrier against infection.

But there's more. That same serving of goji berries has more than 15% of the vitamin C men and women require each day. This vitamin supports your skin so it can help prevent toxins from entering your body, and helps stimulate the production of white blood cells that kill foreign microbes.

Enjoy these chewy, slightly sour fruits as you would raisins. Dried goji berries go great in cookies, trail mix, and cereal. Or just toss back a handful for a quick snack. And don't worry about your dried goji berries going bad any time soon. You can store them in a sealed container for up to a year.

Protect your peepers. Goji berries are a naturally rich source of the antioxidant zeaxanthin, which is particularly important to people in the early stages of age-related macular degeneration (AMD).

That's what researchers discovered after studying 114 adults with this condition. Half of them ate a little less than an ounce of goji berries daily over three months. The rest took a placebo. At the end of the study, the people who ate the goji berries were able to see better and had improvements in their retinas' macular pigment density.

It's important because macular pigment helps protect your eyes from the harmful blue light emitted by the sun and electronic equipment. In fact, the folks who ate the goji berries had three times more zeaxanthin in their blood at the end of the study than they did at the start.

Kitchen hacks

It sure can be disappointing to find your berries covered with white fuzz just a few days after buying them. Try these hacks to keep these tasty treats fresh for longer.

Next time you get home from the market, dunk your berries for 30 seconds in water that's been heated to 125 degrees. This will help prevent mold growth. Remove the berries from the heat bath, and lay them on a towel to dry.

If you'd rather not turn on the stove, you can also stop mold in its tracks with a vinegar soak. Mix 1 part apple cider vinegar to 3 parts water and cover the berries with the liquid for five minutes. Rinse well and dry.

Refrigerate the fruit in a large container lined with paper towels. Leave the lid partially open to allow moisture to escape. Enjoy!

Snack on this to banish belly fat

The number seems to go up each year. Not your age, your waistline. While extra belly fat might bother you because of how it looks, it can actually be dangerous to your health.

That's because excess belly fat isn't limited to a bit of extra padding around your waist. It includes visceral fat that lies deep inside your belly, wraps itself around your vital organs, and is linked to health problems like type 2 diabetes, heart disease, and high blood pressure.

And this is where blueberries come in. Surprising research suggests this fruit contains compounds that reduce belly fat.

That's according to scientists at the University of Michigan who fed obesity-prone rats either a high-fat or low-fat diet. Half of the rats also received blueberry powder with their meals. The rest got a placebo.

At the end of three months, all of the rats who ate the blueberry powder with their meals lost belly fat. They also saw improvements in their triglyceride and cholesterol levels, as well as their sensitivity to insulin. Not so with those on the placebo.

As an added bonus, the rats on the low-fat diet with blueberry powder also lost a significant amount of weight.

So how do you know if your belly fat is a problem? Pull out the tape measure. Health risks from visceral fat are linked to a waist circumference of 35 inches or more for women and 40 inches or more for men.

A closer look
Storing produce

Seems like the price of fresh produce keeps going up and up. But you can avoid paying more by using these money-saving tips.

- Weigh fixed-price, pre-bagged fruits and veggies. Choose the heaviest to get the most bang for your buck.

- Look for deals in discounted grocery stores or farmers markets. Buy only what is in season.

- Don't turn away from slightly bruised or misshapen produce. It's the markdown that counts.

Once you get your groceries home, stretch your dollars even more by shrinking waste. Most fruits and veggies should be stored in your refrigerator's crisper compartments. You can keep your produce fresh for days or even weeks longer by simply placing a clean, dry sponge in the drawers with them to absorb excess moisture.

But store unwashed strawberries and blueberries in their original container in the main section of the fridge. Or pack them loosely in a plastic container lined with paper towels. Leave the lid off to promote proper airflow.

Allow bananas, avocados, melons, peaches, and pears to ripen on the kitchen counter. You should loosely stack potatoes in a cool, dry place that's well ventilated. Leave onions and garlic on the kitchen counter.

These pointers will also help keep produce fresh.

- Bananas ripening too quickly? Wrap the stems in plastic to prevent ethylene gas from spreading to other parts of the fruit.

- Stand trimmed asparagus stems in a glass containing an inch of water. Cover with a plastic bag before refrigerating.

- Never freeze fresh mushrooms. Keep them unwashed and refrigerated in their original packaging. Rinse mushrooms only when you're ready to slice or cook them.

Cherries

Tart traditions: Enhance your memory and sleep time

Where did you set your keys down? When are you supposed to change that water filter, again? And how long has it been since you've actually gotten a full night of sleep? If these questions are running through your head more often than not, you may need a turbo shot of the brain-boosting chemicals found in cherry juice. Drinking this twice a day may help you think clearly, remember more, and sleep better.

Juice up your brain function. If you've ever asked "Pretty please, with a cherry on top," then maybe you know how wonderful this fruit is. But do you know how good it is for you? Cherries are full of natural plant chemicals that work hard to keep your brain working its best, especially if you're a senior.

Researchers at the University of Delaware agree. They split a group of seniors in two groups. One group drank 2 cups of Montmorency tart cherry juice each day for three months and the other drank a placebo. At 12 weeks, the people drinking the cherry juice were more satisfied with their memory than the placebo group. Not only that, but the cherry drinkers also had a 23% improvement when tested on visual memory and the ability to learn new things.

Scientists believe this improvement in brain function is caused by natural plant chemicals — polyphenols, anthocyanins, and melanin — that act as antioxidants in the body. But you won't feel the effects overnight. It can take several weeks for these chemicals to build up in your brain tissues and begin to work.

Drink to a better night's sleep. Less stress, a healthy weight, fewer sick days, a clear mind, and a happy mood. Getting enough sleep could make this your reality. If that sounds like a dream, you're in luck. You may sleep sounder and wake refreshed and ready to face the day when you add cherry juice and cherries to your menu.

You don't have to suffer a restless night. In addition to drinking cherry juice, try these tips for having a deeper sleep. Cut off coffee or soda at midday, and avoid heavy meals one to three hours before bedtime. Create a calming bedtime routine that includes limiting screens and turning down the lights.

When researchers looked into the theory, they found that 2 tablespoons of tart cherry juice concentrate twice a day for a week improved sleep time compared to a non-cherry placebo. The scientists also found that drinking cherry juice increased levels of melatonin — a hormone that regulates your body's natural sleep-wake cycle.

Kick arthritis to the curb with this little red fruit

A standard-sized cherry tree can yield up to a whopping 50 quarts of cherries per season. Good thing, too, since cherries can do more than just help you sleep better. Read on to discover what else this mighty fruit can do.

Tasty treats relieve gouty arthritis pain. Gout is a form of inflammatory arthritis with symptoms that come and go, sneaking up on you when you least expect it. The cause? Uric acid. This substance builds up at the joint, leading to aches and inflammation. After one episode of this intense red hot, burning pain, you'll be searching for ways to avoid another one.

Luckily, preventing another gout attack could be as simple as eating more cherries, say scientists who surveyed the diets of more than 600 people with gout over a year. They found that those who ate cherries over a two-day period had a 35% lower risk of gout attacks than those who didn't.

The researchers believe that cherries' anti-inflammatory activity and ability to decrease uric acid levels make them a powerful tool in gout prevention.

Scale down osteoarthritis inflammation. More than 32 million adults suffer from osteoarthritis, a painful and debilitating disease that causes the padding between joints to wear away. Nonsteroidal anti-inflammatory drugs (NSAIDs) are often prescribed to help treat the inflammation and pain following bone-on-bone friction at the joints. While effective, NSAIDs have many side effects like stomach pain and bleeding. Enter cherry juice — the highly nutritious and delicious drink that can reduce inflammation sans negative and painful side effects.

That's according to researchers who found that drinking cherry juice may help fight osteoarthritis. A small group of women struggling with this painful disease drank 21 ounces of tart cherry juice or a placebo every day for three weeks. The level of CRP, which is a marker of inflammation, in the cherry drinkers' blood decreased.

"With millions of Americans looking for ways to naturally manage pain, it's promising that tart cherries can help, without the possible side effects often associated with arthritis

Want to make your own cherry juice? Pit and stem 6 cups of cherries, then blend them with 3/4 cup of water. Pour the mixture into a strainer, letting the juice fall into a bowl. Place in fridge and drink within three days.

medications," says lead author Dr. Kerry Kuehl. "I'm intrigued by the potential for a real food to offer such a powerful anti-inflammatory benefit — especially for active adults."

So put eating wholesome foods like cherries at the top of your to-do list. After all, reducing inflammation can boost immunity and help your body fight other chronic diseases.

 Kitchen hacks

Don't become one of those customers who eat cherries in the produce section just to see if they're ripe. Instead, follow these tips to choose, store, and prep the perfect cherry every time.

- Pick cherries that are firm, plump, and shiny, with their green stems still attached. Sweet cherries will be dark red in color while Rainier cherries have a yellow to light-red hue.

- The key to keeping cherries fresh is to get them in the refrigerator ASAP. Wait to wash them until just before eating.

- When you're ready to start snacking, remove the stem and the pit. You can use a cherry pitter or a paring knife. Or simply push a metal straw or chopstick through the top of the cherry and gently push the pit out the other side.

The heart-happy snack that packs amazing artery-cleaning power

Tickers come in all sizes, from the microscopic heart of the 0.006-inch fairy fly to the golf cart-sized heart of the blue whale. While yours is closer to the size of your fist, one thing is the same across the board. Without a healthy heart, the body suffers. Happily, cherries contain impressive nutrients that keep your ticker in check.

Score more perks for your blood pressure and cholesterol. The Cherry Marketing Institute has branded the Montmorency tart cherry as "the cherry with more." Extra flavor, exceptional health benefits — no wonder the nonprofit funded a two-phase study to discover just what this delicious little fruit has to offer.

The research, published in the medical journals *Nutrients* and *Food & Function*, put these cherries on top. In the study, one group of adults drank a cup of Montmorency tart cherry juice in the morning and evening each day while the other drank a placebo. After 12 weeks, the tart cherry juice group had decreases in systolic blood pressure and LDL cholesterol compared to the placebo group.

"Our findings suggest that tart cherry juice could be an easy and effective way to add more nutrient-rich fruit to the diet and maintain heart health," says lead researcher Sheau Ching Chai, Ph.D. "We believe the unique nutrient content of Montmorency tart cherries, including the potassium and bioactive compounds, may be contributing factors."

A dose of fiber in every handful to fight heart disease and stroke. One cup of sweet cherries has 3.2 grams of fiber, or 15% of the daily needs for a woman and 11% for a man. It's the soluble fiber, in particular, that acts as a boon to your blood vessels.

This is according to researchers who analyzed results from 31 studies on fiber and heart health. They found that people who ate the highest amount of fiber had up to a 24% lower risk of heart disease and stroke. The reduced risk comes from soluble fiber's ability to lower total cholesterol and the bad, LDL, cholesterol. Soluble fiber limits the cholesterol you absorb from food, keeping it out of your bloodstream and away from the walls of your arteries.

Citrus

A bite of sunshine: 3 reasons to savor citrus

A single citrus plant can have over 60,000 flowers, but only 1% of those will develop into a fruit. It's just one of the interesting facts about this produce with a fragrant, pulpy center. Here's another tidbit that will have you wanting to learn more. Eating just one serving a day could reduce your risk of the following life-threatening conditions.

Keep strokes at bay. While early detection and treatment can help reduce damage from a stroke, adding more vitamin C-rich citrus to your diet can cut your risk of having one in the first place.

Those are the findings of a long-term British study of some 20,000 adults. Researchers found that the people with the highest levels of vitamin C in their blood at the start of the study were nearly half as likely to have a stroke as those with the lowest levels.

Just 1 cup of orange sections provides both men and women with more than 100% of the recommended daily amount of this important vitamin. Grapefruits, lemons, and limes are also loaded with it. So get peeling!

Fight heart disease. Need another reason to add citrus to your diet? A long-term study of health care professionals found that those who ate the most fruits and veggies had a significantly lower risk of developing heart disease than those who ate the least.

And here's the kicker. Produce rich in vitamin C provided the most protection, along with green leafy vegetables. Even one extra serving a day had an effect. So nibble on some kumquats.

This olive-sized citrus is high in vitamin C. Just wash and pop into your mouth whole to take advantage of the sweet-tart taste.

Whittle you middle. Load up on fruits and veggies — including citrus — if you want to avoid the extra pounds that often pile on later in life. That's what researchers discovered after following the diets of 70,000 healthy women over more than a decade.

They found that the participants who increased the amount of produce they ate were much less likely to become obese or have major weight gain. A possible reason why? Fruits and veggies are low in calories and high in fiber, which helps you feel full and satisfied.

Citrus may also help with weight loss. Scientists at the University of Western Ontario discovered that the flavonoids in this fruit shrank the size of fat cells and reversed the obesity in mice that were fed a diet high in fat and cholesterol.

Hate trimming the white, stringy pith from a grapefruit or orange? Here's a neat trick. Use the palm of your hand to roll the fruit around on a table before peeling. This helps to separate the peel and pith from the part you're going to eat.

Banish blood-sugar blues with grapefruit

Grapefruits sure are a healthy addition to any menu. They can boost weight loss as well as help keep blood sugar levels in check — something particularly important for folks who want to remain in good shape.

In a three-month study, obese adults who ate half a grapefruit before breakfast, lunch, and dinner each day saw a significant reduction in their insulin levels, suggesting improvements in their sensitivity to this hormone. That's important because insulin prompts your cells to absorb sugar for energy, thus preventing elevated blood glucose levels that can lead to type 2 diabetes.

Not only that, the participants lost more than 3 1/2 pounds. The scientists say grapefruit — which clocks in at around 75 calories per cup — takes up a lot of room in the belly. That may have caused the participants to eat less at mealtime.

 Watch out

Grapefruit provides lots of fiber and other important nutrients, but it may not be the best choice for everyone.

This fruit and its juices contain compounds that can interfere with the enzymes that break down prescription medications in your digestive system. When this happens, your bloodstream may absorb too much of the drug. This can cause dangerous side effects. Conversely, the medication can also be broken down too quickly, making it less effective.

Here's a list of some types of drugs that can interact with grapefruit.

- anti-anxiety medications
- antihistamines
- blood pressure medications
- blood thinners
- corticosteroids
- organ-transplant rejection medications
- statin drugs to lower cholesterol

Always talk with your doctor about your medications and how they might interact with this fruit.

2 juicy secrets for optimum health

What nutrient comes to mind when you think of citrus? Vitamin C often stands out, but it's not the only contender. Other powerful compounds in these fruits also have significant health benefits.

Hesperidin fights off COVID-19. Four of the seven coronaviruses that infect people usually cause mild to moderate cold-like symptoms. But over the past 20 years, the other three have caused widespread disease. The most recent coronavirus is the highly contagious COVID-19.

Fortunately, recent research has found that a powerful chemical found only in citrus fruits may be useful in preventing COVID-19. It's called hesperidin, and scientists say it may help fight the virus by preventing it from entering and infecting human cells.

Of course, these findings are preliminary. But we do know that citrus fruits have other benefits for respiratory illnesses. One large orange has over 100% of your daily vitamin C needs — a nutrient that may help cut the time it takes to recover from viral infections like the common cold.

Phytochemicals lower cancer risk. If you like green tea, you're in luck. This beverage is loaded with catechins, a substance that helps protect your cells from free radicals. Those are unstable molecules that, over the long term, damage your cells and may play a role in the development of cancer.

The problem, however, is that most of the catechins get destroyed during digestion. That greatly reduces the amount your cells can absorb. But here's the good news. Lab studies have found that lemon juice increases the availability of catechins in green tea by up to 80%. So don't forget to add a bit of this juice into your next cup of green tea.

After lemon juice, the next best stabilizing powers were orange, lime, and grapefruit juices. Researchers are still learning how citrus pulled this off, but say the fruit's phytochemicals may prevent the damage to catechins that normally occurs during digestion.

Bright idea

Yikes! Last night's spaghetti sauce has stained your new Tupperware container an orange-red. You could just add it to the stack of your other tainted containers. Or, you can put that lemon on your counter to use.

Try this task on a sunny day. The power from the lemon and the sun's heat work together to get your plastic bowls sparkling clean.

Cut the lemon in half and rub the fleshy part over the stains, squeezing out the juice as you go. Or, you could soak a dishcloth in the lemon juice and scrub the container that way. Place the dish in direct sunlight for at least 30 minutes before rinsing and then washing with dish soap and water. Dry with a clean cloth. Your plastic container is as good as new!

Zest for life — feast your way to better skin

Bleeding gums, loose teeth, weakness, and loss of appetite — all signs of scurvy. This was once the reality for sailors who went for long periods without any vitamin C. If only it were possible to go back in time and tell these mariners to load up on citrus.

Fortunately, scurvy is relatively rare these days. But snacking on this fruit is still a great idea, especially if you're after healthy and youthful skin.

Heal wounds with ease. Not eating enough vitamin C can make scratches, sores, and other wounds more difficult to heal. That's because your body needs this nutrient to create collagen, a fibrous protein necessary for your skin's structural support.

Aging, meanwhile, causes a decline in the vitamin C in the outer layers of your skin. That's why it's so important that older folks get enough — 75 milligrams a day for women and 90 milligrams for men. Just one cup of pink and red grapefruit sections provides 85 milligrams.

Say goodbye to wrinkles. Scientists surveyed over 4,000 middle-aged women, comparing the nutrients in their diets with signs of aging skin. They found that the women who ate or drank higher amounts of vitamin C tended to have fewer wrinkles and more hydrated skin.

Researchers point to vitamin C's antioxidant powers that help protect the skin from sun damage. And of course, all that collagen production helps to give your skin strength and elasticity.

Here's an idea. Want to get even more vitamin C when you're eating your morning grapefruit? Add some kiwi, guava, cantaloupe, or papaya to the mix. Although they're not technically citrus, these fruits also contain high amounts of this nutrient.

Name that orange! The inside scoop on the top varieties

No doubt about it. The sweet, seedless navel orange is perfect for snacking or tossing into a lunchbox. And it's one of the most popular fruits around, easily recognized by a belly-button like mark on one end.

Read on for other types of oranges you'll want to consider next time you're at the market.

Valencia. This thin-skinned orange is the perfect choice when it comes to making homemade orange juice. Valencia oranges grow in California and Florida and are harvested between March and July.

Blood orange. Unique for their bold-red flesh, blood oranges tend to be smaller than other oranges and have a sweet-tart flavor that further sets them apart. You can find blood oranges from November to March, which makes them delicious additions to winter desserts.

Cara cara. This fruit has pinkish-red flesh, a sweet flavor, and low acidity. It also has fewer seeds than many other oranges, and goes great in a salad. The state of California harvests cara cara oranges from December to April.

Clementine. Small, seedless, and easy to peel, clementines are perfect for snacking. The white pith comes off easily, leaving only sweet flesh behind. You'll find these in peak condition between November and January.

Refrigerating your oranges — and other citrus fruits — in the crisper drawer will extend their shelf life. Return them to room temperature before peeling. This allows the fruit to regain its juiciness.

Blast blood pressure with this breakfast staple

If you're hoping to see the magic numbers 120/80 when you place the blood pressure cuff on your arm, start your day with a glass of orange juice. This popular breakfast drink can help turn arteries into wide-open spaces, and may even lower your blood pressure in just four weeks.

Scientists discovered this after testing the beverage on a group of overweight, but otherwise healthy, men. The researchers learned compounds in orange juice caused the men's diastolic blood pressure — that's the second number in the reading — to drop by 5.5 points. How much did they drink to see these results? Two cups of juice a day for four weeks.

Lead author of the study Christine Morand attributes the results, in part, to the antioxidant hesperidin's ability to widen blood vessels. This promotes blood flow, which lowers blood pressure.

Figs

Snack on this for bone-building power

Was it really an apple that Eve plucked from the tree of knowledge? Some scholars have suggested that the forbidden fruit was actually a fig. No matter, there's no need to forbid the fig from your diet, especially if it's strong bones you're after.

Magnesium. Over half of the magnesium in your body is stored in your bones, making this mineral essential for combating osteoporosis. It's involved in bone formation and it also has a say in how much vitamin D, another bone-building nutrient, your body uses. A quarter-cup of dried figs, or three fresh figs, has 6% of the recommended magnesium for men and 8% for women.

Calcium. Not into gulping down cup after cup of milk? Eat figs to give your bones the calcium boost they need. A quarter-cup of dried figs meets 5% of the daily calcium needs for folks over 70. Almost all of the calcium your body absorbs will go straight to your bones to keep up with growth, repair, and the prevention of the bone-breaking disease osteoporosis.

Potassium. You don't need to rely on bananas to get your daily dose of potassium for healthy bones. This essential mineral, found in many fruits and vegetables including figs, may help neutralize acid in your body that contributes to bone loss.

In a recent study, Korean researchers found that women who ate the most potassium had a 32% reduced risk of lower back osteoporosis compared to women who ate the least. This same effect wasn't seen in the men, but other research has found that eating more potassium-rich foods is associated with higher bone mineral density in both men and women. The denser your bones are, the less likely they are to break.

Just a quarter-cup of dried figs serves up 253 milligrams of potassium, or 10% of the daily value for women over 50 and 7% for men of the same age. Smear some fig jam on toast or serve dried figs alongside goat cheese and crackers for an impressive appetizer sure to help keep your bones strong and healthy.

Soothe your stomach with a sweet snack

If your visit to the porcelain throne is anything but comfortable, you might find relief down the dried fruit or produce aisle. After all, figs are a great source of fiber.

In fact, you'll get about 4 grams of fiber from three fresh figs or five dried figs. That's at least 12% of the daily recommendations for men over 50 and 17% for women of the same age. From constipation to more complicated irritable bowel syndrome (IBS), your bowels will thank you for snacking on this fiber-filled fruit.

Ditch constipation. Have trouble clearing your pipes? You're in good company — 20% of people experience constipation. But don't worry, relief could be sitting right there on your pantry shelf. Researchers in Korea think figs may be the key to helping you easily answer nature's call.

After eight weeks of eating fig paste — the equivalent of about six fresh figs — every day, people with constipation had improvements in their symptoms compared to the placebo group. The fig group had softer, more comfortable bowel movements, and food traveled through their digestive systems more quickly than before.

Ease IBS. Bloating, stomach pain, discomfort. For people with IBS, this isn't just a bad day, but a constant part of life. To see if figs could go to bat for adults who suffered from IBS with constipation, researchers tried it out.

For four months, participants ate 45 grams of — or almost six — dried figs with a glass of water twice a day. They reported improvements in the frequency of pain, bloating, stool hardness, and bowel movements compared to the control group who stuck to their normal diets.

These results are not surprising considering that both the insoluble and soluble fiber in figs can help relieve constipation. The soluble kind helps add bulk to stool while insoluble fiber speeds food along through your digestive tract.

✕ Kitchen hacks

The season for fresh figs is incredibly short with a small window in early summer and another in early fall. If you're lucky enough to snag this fruit while it's fresh, choose figs that are free from blemishes and soft to gentle pressure. Keep them at room temperature to use immediately, or store them in the fridge for two to seven days.

The peel is edible, but not everyone likes its flavor or texture. Easily remove it with a vegetable peeler or cut the fig in half and scoop the inside out with a spoon. Fresh figs pair well with cheeses like goat or feta and can be cooked to intensify their natural sweetness and flavor.

If you miss the window for fresh fruit, dried figs are available any time of year on supermarket shelves. Dice and sprinkle them on your oatmeal, yogurt, salads, or muffins for a sweet nutrient boost.

A closer look
Exotic fruits

Are you feeling bored with apples, pears, and even oranges? Change things up and get a little more "exotic" by trying fruit traditionally grown in tropical regions worldwide. Thanks to modern transportation, you'll only have to travel as far as a well-stocked supermarket to pick up an exotic fruit.

Be aware that some of these fruits are difficult to keep fresh and cost a pretty penny more than their homegrown relatives. Transportation, temperature control during travel, and treatments to keep produce pests from hopping borders are a few reasons you could pay more at the market.

But don't let the price deter you. The flavor, nutrition, and fun of trying new foods can be worth it. Here are several exotic fruits to try if you happen to see them on your next grocery trip.

Jackfruit. With a texture similar to shredded meat, this tropical fruit is popular for plant-based meals. Besides a good option for vegan pulled "pork," jackfruit has a sweet, mellow taste that works well in stews, stir-fries, and fruit salads.

You'll most likely find it in the canned fruit or international aisle, frozen, or with other meat substitutes. It's a great source of potassium, vitamin C, and several B vitamins.

Lychee. This fruit, which is native to China, is in season from late spring to early fall. Choose lychees that are at least 1 inch in diameter and have a bright pinkish-red skin. You'll want to peel the hard, bumpy husk and remove the inedible pit before biting into the sweet, white fruit.

Lychees are extremely low in sodium and cholesterol and a fantastic source of vitamin C. Eat this fruit on its own, or combine it with other tropical fruits. You can also add lychees to curries, salads, and desserts. Mmm.

Mango. The ripe fruit can be any combination of red, yellow, orange, and green. You'll know it's ready to eat when it's slightly soft and fragrant. Ripe mangoes keep in the fridge for up to five days. Enjoy them in smoothies, homemade salsa, or topped on yogurt for an extra dose of folate and vitamins A, C, and E.

One cup of sliced mango has just 107 calories and provides 3 grams of fiber. So enjoy!

Papaya. Cube up some papaya and add it to your fruit salad, water, smoothie, or salsa for a tropical twist. A cup of papaya has around 100% of your daily vitamin C needs and only 62 calories.

Choose one with skin that's tight, smooth, free from dark spots, and slightly soft. To eat, just slice it in half, remove the seeds, and peel the skin or scoop out the sweet flesh with a spoon. If you want to use this fruit beyond snacking, puree it for your next marinade. Papaya has an enzyme called papain, which breaks down muscle fibers, making it a natural meat tenderizer.

Passion fruit. This purple fruit fits a lot of flavor and nutrients in a small package. Each fruit has only 17 calories and contains 2 grams of fiber — 9% of the daily needs for women and 6% for men.

To eat a passion fruit, slice open the hard outer rind and scoop out the juicy flesh and seeds. The pulp and seeds are edible, but you'll want to toss the rind along with the bitter white coating inside it.

While the fruit is good enough to eat on its own, try adding it to yogurt and salads. Or strain the seeds out and use the juice to flavor your water.

Star fruit. This funky-looking fruit is good for more than adding curb appeal to your fruit salad. The slightly tart but deliciously sweet flavor tastes like a combination of pineapple, plums, and lemon. One cup has only 33 calories and over 40% of your daily vitamin C needs.

You can eat every part of the star fruit. It interacts with certain medications, though, so ask your pharmacist first.

Grapes

Vine and dine time: Here's to eating right for better health

Grapes are one of the world's largest fruit crops, with some 75 million tons produced each year. Whether you enjoy them dried into raisins, as a juice, or just straight from the fridge, grapes provide a slew of health benefits — including the ability to lower blood pressure and protect against cancer. Here's what else they can do.

Keep diabetes at bay. Scientists studied the diets of almost 190,000 health care professionals over several decades. They found that those who ate at least three servings of whole fruits per week had a reduced risk of developing type 2 diabetes. Grapes, in particular, were highlighted for their health benefits.

Researchers think this fruit may lower the chances of getting diabetes because some types — including red and black grapes — have high levels of anthocyanins.

Scientists say these plant compounds may decrease the amount of glucose that the liver produces. In addition, both red and white grapes contain resveratrol, a plant compound that may increase insulin sensitivity.

So load up on grapes next time you're in the produce aisle. They're relatively cheap and you can get them year-round at any grocery store. When you get home, toss a bunch into the freezer. The fruit will taste sweeter in a few hours because the sugar in them will crystallize.

Cholesterol gets the kibosh. Eating lots of unhealthy fats can send your cholesterol through the roof. That's one of the reasons it's not a good idea to eat a lot of fast food. Since high cholesterol is a major risk factor for heart disease and stroke, you'll want to choose the right foods to keep your numbers in check.

That's where red grapes come in. Scientists studied adults with high cholesterol and found that those who ate a little more than 3 cups of red grapes daily over two months saw significant improvements in both total and LDL cholesterol levels.

LDL is often called the "bad" cholesterol because it causes fatty buildup in your arteries.

Red grapes are particularly high in fiber and powerful antioxidant plant compounds called polyphenols. Scientists believe the two work together to limit your body's ability to absorb cholesterol.

Juice up brain power. Grape skins can be difficult to chew, especially if you're missing teeth or have loose-fitting dentures. But that doesn't mean you have to miss out on this fruit's brain-boosting powers.

Researchers studied the diets of almost 2,000 older adults over a decade and found that those who drank a refreshing glass of fruit or vegetable juice three times a week had a 76% lower risk of getting Alzheimer's disease than those who drank juice less than once a week. Having it just once or twice a week slashed their risk of this common form of dementia by 16%.

One reason why grape juice might help? It contains quercetin, which researchers say protects nerve cells in the brain from toxins. This plant pigment also reduces inflammation, which is linked to Alzheimer's disease.

Jam up arthritis pain with pectin

Ouch! Your arthritis has kicked in and your knees are stiff and achy. Instead of reaching for painkillers, try this home remedy.

Folks with arthritis swear by a mixture of grape juice and liquid pectin — a natural thickening agent used to make jams and jellies. While there are no scientific studies backing this treatment, experts explain that pectin regulates fluid in and out of cells. That's important because arthritis pain is often caused by the buildup of fluid between joints.

Grape juice has anti-inflammatory properties, making it the perfect addition to pectin. So when your joints begin to bother you, mix 3 ounces of purple grape juice with 2 teaspoons of liquid pectin. Drink up to three times a day until the pain eases.

Grape expectations — boost your bones by the bunch

Osteoporosis. It means porous bones, a condition characterized by a loss of calcium and other minerals in your skeleton. Known as a silent disease, many people have no symptoms until they suffer a life-altering fracture.

Staying active with weight-bearing exercises like walking, dancing, and stair climbing can help keep your frame strong. So can eating a healthy diet. While foods high in calcium and vitamin D might be the first to pop into your mind when you think of bone-strengthening fare, vitamin K is also essential. And grapes are a tasty way to fit this nutrient in.

You'll want to make sure you get enough of this vitamin, particularly if you're an older adult. That's because this nutrient can increase bone mineral density in people with osteoporosis and reduce their risk of fractures. How? For starters, vitamin K activates proteins needed for bone formation and mineralization. It also helps your body retain more calcium, which is so necessary for bone health.

Just 1 cup of red or green grapes has 22 micrograms (mcg) of vitamin K. That's nearly a quarter of the 90 mcg women need each day and almost 20% of the 120 mcg that men require daily.

Suddenly increasing the amount of vitamin K you get each day could lessen the effect of blood thinners you might take for a heart condition. That's because vitamin K plays a key role in helping blood to clot. Talk to your doctor before making such changes to your diet.

Along with grapes, you can find vitamin K in soybeans and leafy greens like kale, spinach, and collards. Prunes and kiwis are also good sources.

Age-proof your vision with this popular fruit

Although age-related vision problems are certainly more common in folks over 50, they aren't inevitable. In fact, you can improve the chances your eyes won't need glasses, contact lenses, surgery, or medicine of any kind as you get older. Just reach for grapes.

But first, some background. How you see the world hinges on your retina. It's the part of your eye that houses millions of cells, called photoreceptors, that convert light into electrical signals. In order to make sense of what you're seeing, the retina sends this information to your brain via an information highway known as the optic nerve.

When damage occurs to the retina, it's often caused by oxidative stress. That's a condition caused by an imbalance of harmful molecules called free radicals and the antioxidants that neutralize them.

Oxidative stress can lead to all sorts of eye problems, including age-related macular degeneration, glaucoma, and diabetic retinopathy.

Now on to the best part. The antioxidants in grapes work like superheroes when it comes to limiting the damage caused by free radicals. Scientists found that grapes' vision-protecting powers included the preservation of both retinal thickness and the health of photoreceptor cells despite high levels of oxidative stress.

The researchers attribute the results to the fact that grapes are packed with vitamin C, vitamin K, and beta carotene — all antioxidants that rid the body of harmful molecules. Although this was an animal study, the scientists believe the results build on growing evidence that eating grapes can benefit eye health.

 Bright idea

Oh, the plans you had last week for that bag of grapes in the crisper drawer. Only now they're getting mushy. Instead of tossing your sad "almost bad" grapes, revive them with these tips.

- Roast at 420 degrees for 20 minutes or until the skins start to split. Once cooled, refrigerate the fruit in an airtight container. Add to salads or just toss back as a quick snack.

- Dehydrate to make raisins. Blanch the grapes in boiling water for 30 seconds, then transfer to an ice bath. Cut the grapes in half and lay them in a single layer on a cookie sheet. Bake at 180 degrees for 18 to 24 hours, rotating halfway through. Store in an airtight container in the pantry.

- Freeze to use as ice cubes that won't water down your drink. Or mix frozen grapes with a little lemon juice and water in the blender for a refreshing slushie.

Melons

Tap into wondrous watermelon for a trimmer, healthier body

The days are long and the sun is hot. But don't fret. A wedge of ice-cold, juicy watermelon will revive you. This fruit is 92% water, perfect for keeping you hydrated in the summer heat.

But that's not all you'll gain. Watermelon also provides other awesome health benefits.

Lose weight deliciously. Here's a sweet way to fill up and slim down. In a recent study, overweight and obese adults ate either 2 cups of diced watermelon or six low-fat cookies each day for a month. Both snacks had about 90 calories.

At the end of the study, the people who ate the watermelon lost weight and saw decreases in their body mass index. The cookie eaters, meanwhile, experienced increases in both. To make matters worse, their blood pressure also rose.

Watermelon's staying power was key to the participants' weight loss. Those who ate the fruit said they didn't feel hungry for up to two hours after the snack. And the cookie eaters? They were ready to head to the fridge after just 20 minutes.

Of course, the watermelon weighed more and took up more belly room than the cookies. That likely meant it took longer to chew and digest, which also improves feelings of being satisfied.

So eat more watermelon — and don't forget the black seeds. They're loaded with magnesium and are a rich source of protein and iron. Toast them in the oven at 325 degrees for about 15 minutes and add to salads or trail mix.

Keep your ticker in tiptop shape. Ever heard of lycopene? If not, you'll want to learn about this heart-healthy antioxidant that gives red fruits like watermelon their color.

While there's no set amount of lycopene you should get, Dr. Edward Giovannucci, a professor of nutrition and epidemiology at the Harvard School of Public Health, recommends getting at least 10 milligrams (mg) a day. That's easy to do when it comes to watermelon. Just 2 cups of this diced fruit has nearly 14 mg.

The first recorded watermelon harvest took place nearly 5,000 years ago in Egypt. This fruit was so beloved for keeping folks hydrated in the hot desert climate that mourners buried King Tut with watermelon seeds. Why? To provide him nourishment in the afterlife.

Here's the really neat part. Researchers analyzed the results of six studies on lycopene and found that a little over 12 mg per day of this antioxidant was enough to lower systolic blood pressure — that's the higher and top number on your reading — by an average of 5 points over eight weeks.

Scientists believe lycopene lowers blood pressure by reducing oxidative stress. That could indirectly stimulate the production of nitric oxide in the blood vessels, causing them to widen. That means your heart doesn't have to work as hard to pump blood.

Oh — don't toss out your watermelon rind. It has lots of water and nutrients. Peel off the green skin and go ahead and pickle, stir-fry, or juice the rind. You can even eat it raw.

Kitchen hacks

Follow these tips to pick the perfect melon every time.

- **Cantaloupe.** Look for a firm, pale melon that's free of blemishes and heavy for its size. It should have a smooth bottom with a slight indentation. Ripe cantaloupes have a slightly sweet and musky aroma, and the seeds inside will rattle when you shake the fruit.

- **Honeydew.** The rind should be a creamy yellow color. It should feel firm but give a little bit when you press into it. Smell the melon and look for a sweet, lightly floral scent. Drum your fingers lightly over the fruit and listen for a dull thud.

- **Watermelon.** Check for a yellow or orange-yellow spot on the rind. It's a sign that the fruit was left to ripen before being picked. Rap the side of the melon with your knuckles — it should have a hollow sound. Look for a dull rind that gives slightly under pressure.

First on the honey-'dew' list: Get more potassium

You can thank your kidneys for creating urine from the waste and excess water in your blood. But sometimes things don't always go as planned, and minerals and salts build up in these bean-shaped organs. Next thing you know, you've been diagnosed with kidney stones.

But help is on the way. A review of three landmark studies found that people whose diets included high levels of potassium were 33% to 56% less likely to develop kidney stones. One possible reason? Sometimes stones form when the acid levels in urine grow too high. Potassium is an alkaline that neutralizes the acids.

And that's where honeydew melon comes in. A little over 6 ounces of this fruit contains 404 milligrams of potassium. That's 12% of what a man should get daily, and 16% of what a woman requires. So feel free to eat up. That same amount of honeydew has only 64 calories.

Can't top cantaloupe — 2 surprising health benefits

Legend has it that Christopher Columbus introduced cantaloupe seeds to the New World sometime after his second voyage to the Caribbean in late 1493. The fruit has since become wildly popular, and the average American eats nearly 9 pounds of it a year. The best part? Cantaloupes are not only sweet and juicy — they're chock-full of nutrients necessary for good health.

Keep muscles strong with vitamin C. It hardly gets better when it comes to cantaloupes and vitamin C. Just half a medium-sized melon provides seniors with more than 100% of the recommended daily amount. This vitamin acts as an antioxidant and helps keep your immune system in tiptop shape. It can also help you remain independent as you age.

A recent British study of 13,000 people between the ages of 42 and 82 found that those who got plenty of vitamin C also had the best muscle mass. People tend to lose muscle strength as they get older, which can limit their ability to do routine activities.

Vitamin C helps defend cells from harmful rogue molecules called free radicals, says lead researcher Ailsa Welch, Ph.D. "Unopposed these free radicals can contribute to the destruction of muscle, thus speeding up age-related decline," she says.

Beta carotene keeps breast cancer at bay. Cantaloupe's orange hue comes from beta carotene, a plant pigment known for its antioxidant properties. Your body converts this nutrient into vitamin A, which it uses to keep your vision sharp, your skin healthy, and your immune system strong.

As it turns out, this antioxidant does even more. A decades-long study of female health care professionals found that those who had high levels of beta carotene in their blood were significantly less likely to develop breast cancer than those with low levels.

Luckily, cantaloupe can get you well on your way to getting more of this nutrient. A little more than 6 ounces of this fruit — about what can fit into a cup — contains 3,575 micrograms of beta carotene. That makes it an excellent source of this important nutrient.

Want to get more of this fruit into your diet? Cantaloupes are a perfect addition to both lettuce and fruit salads. You can also enjoy them in salsas, or mixed with banana, yogurt, and crushed nuts.

Curb arthritis pain with bitter melon

Did you know bitter melon isn't really a melon? It's a member of the gourd family, which includes pumpkins, squash, and cucumbers. Still, you'll want to try this healthy staple of Asian cuisine — especially if you're battling arthritis pain.

In one study, adults with knee osteoarthritis took 1,500 milligrams of bitter melon supplements three times a day over 12 weeks. After that time, they reported significant improvements in their pain and quality of life. The researchers aren't sure why this fruit had such an effect, but bitter melon's anti-inflammatory powers may be responsible.

One thing though. This type of melon tastes, well, bitter. You can remove some of the harsh flavor by salting the fruit and draining the fluids before rinsing and stir-frying. You can also find bitter melon extract at the supermarket.

Prunes

2 nutrients that back your brain and bones

Does the thought of prunes bring up images of your grandparents? Well, this "old folk" food may actually help keep you from getting "old folk" diseases like memory loss and osteoporosis. With benefits like that, people young and old should be snacking on this tasty dried fruit.

An unexpected duo supports your mind. With age comes wisdom, but what good is knowing things if you can't remember them? Age-related memory loss might seem inevitable, but it may not be if prunes have a say in the matter.

The reason comes down to two nutrients. Slipping memory is linked to a drop in antioxidant levels in the brain as well as not getting enough of a mineral called boron. Eating prunes can help you with both.

Boron does more than protect your memory. To keep important skills like hand-eye coordination, manual dexterity, and attention well into your golden years, be sure you eat prunes each day. The boron in them is one of the many minerals that help keep your body young.

They're packed with phenolic acids, anthocyanins, and other flavonoids, which are known to act as antioxidants. Plus they also contain a hefty amount of boron.

Tag-team your skeleton to preserve your strength. With age, also comes the risk that your bones will break down faster than they can build themselves back up — leading to an increased risk of osteoporosis and fractures. This is especially true for women in the first 10 years after menopause, when the most bone is lost.

In a study, one group of women ate 100 grams of prunes daily — approximately 10 prunes — while the other group had a comparable amount of dried apples. Both groups took 500 milligrams of calcium and 10 micrograms of vitamin D each day. After a year, both dried fruits showed bone-protective effects, but the women in the prune group had better bone mineral density in their spines and forearms.

The researchers say that prunes may improve bone mineral density in postmenopausal women by suppressing the rate of bone breakdown, which often outpaces bone growth as you get older. With high levels of antioxidants, they're the perfect fruit to combat free radicals that chip away at bone. The boron in prunes also helps your body retain calcium so that it can be used for bone growth and maintenance.

The sweet cure for constipation

What goes in must come out, but what happens when the coming out part is painful, hard, and infrequent? Constipation isn't the same for everyone. Signs of this condition show up in many forms.

- less than three bowel movements per week
- straining when you go or having hard or lumpy stool
- feeling as though your bowel movements are incomplete

Whether you experience any of these occasionally or frequently, adding prunes to your diet could make your time in the bathroom more productive.

Perhaps that's no surprise, given the prune's reputation for being a laxative. But how many should you eat to get things moving again? In one study, a group of adults on a low-fiber diet ate eight prunes and a cup of water each day for four weeks. Their stool weight and frequency increased compared to a group that drank just the water.

Prunes are a powerhouse at keeping your digestive system running smoothly for a number of reasons. For starters, eight prunes have more than 5 grams of fiber, which is over 24% of the recommended daily value for women and 17% of the daily value for men. This extra fiber helps increase the volume and moisture of stool, making it easier to pass.

And it's not just the fiber either. Prunes also contain a sugar alcohol known as sorbitol, which travels through your system undigested, pulling water into your stool with a laxative-like effect.

 Kitchen hacks

Prunes are easy to come by. But if you want to cut out the preservatives, or happen to have a surplus of plums on your hands, you can make your own.

- Wash and slice the plums in half, removing the pit. Place them flesh-side down directly on the oven rack with a foil-lined pan underneath to catch the juices.

- Set your oven as low as it can go, 200 degrees or lower if possible. Check the plums every few hours until they are wrinkly and mostly dried out — often eight to 12 hours.

- If your prunes are still somewhat soft, store them in the refrigerator for up to a month or in the freezer for 12 to 18 months to prevent mold. If you've fully dehydrated them — so that they look and feel like a raisin — you can keep them in an airtight container at room temperature for up to a year.

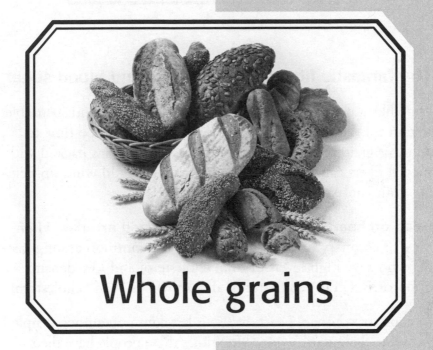

Whole grains

Barley

The fantastic fiber for cholesterol and blood sugar

Dine like a pharaoh. That's right, barley played an indispensable role in the diets of ancient Egyptians. And it may be time to add this grain to your own meal plan. After all, it's packed with special fibers called cereal beta glucans that could wind up helping your cholesterol and blood sugar levels.

Head off heart disease by tackling clogged arteries. High rates of coronary heart disease (CHD) are common among people who have high levels of total cholesterol and low-density lipoprotein (LDL) cholesterol, also known as "bad" cholesterol.

In contrast, coronary heart disease is less common among people with low cholesterol levels. Oftentimes these people have diets that are low in fat and high in fibrous foods, like fruits and grains. Some research suggests that adding soluble fiber to diets already low in saturated fat and cholesterol may lower the risk of CHD.

That's where barley steps in. Research shows that it helps lower levels of dangerous LDL cholesterol, which can gum up your blood vessels. Scientists attribute its benefits to the soluble fiber beta glucan. This is the same fiber responsible for making oats the poster child of heart health. But barley has a leg up since it contains more protein and fewer calories.

Fiber-filled barley is your blood sugar solution. One reason dietary guidelines recommend fiber in your meals is because it's associated with the prevention of chronic conditions like type 2 diabetes. Research suggests that beta glucans are one of the best types of fiber for warding off diabetes because of their ability to lower glucose response after meals.

Beta glucans are viscous fibers, meaning they thicken when mixed with fluid, and stall digestion. This in turn slows the absorption of glucose into your bloodstream.

 Boost the benefits

Some grains lose their fiber after being processed because it's only present in their outer layer. Barley doesn't have the same problem. It has fiber throughout the whole kernel. That means even products like barley flour will contain the beta glucan soluble fiber that gives this grain many of its great health benefits.

All it takes to get barley into your diet is a simple swap. Trade your rice and other processed grains for this alternative. Brown and fortified white rice have some helpful nutrients, but overall barley has more to offer.

Top off your energy tank with this go-to grain

Tired and sluggish? Barley is one kind of food that could give you more energy. That's thanks to the powerhouse nutrients it contains. Find out about some of the top contributors.

Carve out space for complex carbs. Grains like barley are excellent sources of complex carbohydrates. This type of carb breaks down more slowly than simple carbs, so it provides energy to your body slower and is less likely to be converted into fat. Getting enough carbs is vital to fueling your body so your muscles and brain can stay active.

Iron out your energy problems. Low iron levels can make you feel fatigued, even if you don't have anemia, a lack of the iron-rich red blood cells needed to move oxygen across your body.

This essential mineral isn't just important because of its role in oxygen transport, though. It also has a role in creating your body's energy source, adenosine triphosphate, known more familiarly as ATP. A cup of hulled barley swoops in with 83% of the iron you need each day.

Come out ahead with manganese. An essential metal, manganese is a must-have for regulating your energy. It helps create and activate enzymes, which are proteins that speed up the chemical reactions happening in your body.

Manganese also participates in the breakdown of glucose, part of the energy production process. Deficiencies in manganese are uncommon, but you can make sure you get all of your daily needs in a cup of hulled of barley.

If you have celiac disease or are sensitive to gluten, barley is not for you. This grain contains gluten proteins that can make you feel ill. Barley may even be hiding behind names that could slip past your radar. So check for ingredients that include "malt," like malt syrup, dextrimaltose, and maltose.

The nutrient that puts the "b" in barley. Each of the eight B vitamins has their own special role. These vitamins help convert food into energy, on top of other tasks like creating new blood cells. Take vitamin B1 — also called thiamine — for example. Because it helps transform food into fuel, fatigue is a common symptom of a deficiency.

Since B vitamins rely on one another, it's essential to power up your diet with all of them. Fortunately, barley is rich in a variety of B vitamins, including thiamine, niacin, riboflavin, and B6.

Kitchen hacks

Hulled barley versus pearl barley — the big difference is simply how they've been processed. The hulled kind has only the tough outermost husk removed, and it's a whole grain with loads of fiber and nutrients. Pearl or pearled barley is more processed, with the husks and bran layers removed. It's still good for you but is less nutritious than its hulled peer.

If you know how to cook brown rice, you can cook barley. The two processes are very similar, and best of all, easy. Pearl barley will cook more quickly than the hulled version, but you can prepare both on the stovetop.

Improve your basic barley by allowing it to steam after you strain it. Let it rest covered in the pot with the heat off for about 10 minutes. You can also cook barley in vegetable or chicken broth instead of water for extra flavor.

Fill up on these fluffy mixed grains to trim your waistline

White rice might be tasty, but too much of it could make you gain weight. Barley makes an excellent substitute. You don't even have to make this a complete swap to see benefits.

One study shows that simply eating a meal with white rice and barley mixed together can control your appetite better than white rice alone. In addition, participants who ate the mixed grains devoured less at later meals.

Researchers say barley encourages the release of hormones that make you feel full. That's a step in the right direction for way-laying weight gain.

You can make this dish easily at home, too. Called "mugi gohan" in Japan, it literally means barley rice. Swap white rice for brown rice for a healthier twist. Rinse the rice and barley in a sieve and pour them together into a pot of boiling water. Cook on low heat for about 45 minutes. Remove from heat and let it sit for 10 minutes before removing the lid and fluffing with a fork.

The soft rice paired with chewy barley gives this recipe an interesting texture. You can experiment with your ratio of rice to barley, but 3-to-1 is a good place to start.

Barley is one of six foods you should be eating regularly if you're over 55. Also feast on sweet potatoes, salmon, yogurt, broccoli, and apples. The key here is having a balanced diet from various food groups so you get all the major nutrients you need, from vitamin C to omega-3s.

Bright idea

Love to cozy up with a cup of tea? Roasted barley tea is popular in Korea, China, and Japan, and could be your next favorite, whether you want a steaming mug or cool glass.

Roasted barley infuses a smoky, nutty flavor into the tea, but it's milder in taste than green and black varieties. Add a splash of fruit juice or a little sweetener to adjust the flavor to your liking.

To brew, buy roasted barley or make your own by toasting barley in a dry skillet over medium heat for about 10 minutes until golden. Pour the grain into boiling water, with 1 tablespoon of barley for every 4 cups of water. Let it simmer for 20 minutes.

With every sip, you'll get a mouthful of antioxidants, which may help fight a number of chronic conditions. Traditionally, people also drink it for digestive relief, sleep problems, and oral health.

Brown rice

Darker rice, healthier life: Effortless menu swap sinks your odds of diabetes

Rice has been a staple food for at least 5,000 years. But modern science has found that too much of the white variety can raise your risk of diabetes. As a central feature of many diets, simply cutting it out is easier said than done. So instead of putting rice on the chopping block, try making a switch to brown rice. You'll be glad you did, and here's why.

White rice is cheap with a long shelf life but doesn't bring much nutritional value. To make white rice, the grains undergo refining and milling. During this process, the rice bran is removed, which eliminates much of the nutrients. White rice also has a high glycemic index, which means it can quickly cause a hike in your blood sugar. Too much glucose in your blood increases your risk of diabetes.

Research suggests that replacing white rice with brown rice may drop your chances of developing type 2 diabetes. That's because brown rice doesn't spike blood sugar levels. It's less processed and so still contains the fiber-rich outer layer that slows down digestion and the release of sugar into your bloodstream.

Another benefit of fiber is that it can make you feel fuller, longer. This could help protect against weight gain, which is another factor that heightens your diabetes risk. Research backs this up. One study on overweight women even showed that substituting white rice with brown rice increased weight loss, particularly around the waist and hips.

Bright idea

Who says you have to cook your rice? Try these clever household tricks using uncooked grains.

- Sprinkle a little into your saltshaker to suck out excess moisture and keep the salt from clumping up and clogging the holes.

- Cover unripe fruit with rice in a container to speed up the ripening process. This tip is best for harder-skinned fruits, like mangoes and avocados.

- Pour half a cup of rice into your blender and give it a quick run, pulsing for up to two minutes, to sharpen the blades.

- Use it to scrub heavy grime off of narrow vases and bottles. Mix two spoonfuls of rice in the container with warm water and liquid soap. Leave this concoction to soak for 15 minutes, then cover the opening and give it a good shake. Empty, rinse, and you're all set.

The best tricks to lower arsenic levels

Arsenic is a scary-sounding chemical, and for good reason. The inorganic kind that comes from soil and groundwater can create symptoms like nausea, vomiting, and dehydration if you eat or drink large doses. Exposure may even increase your cancer risk over the long term. That's why it pays to be picky about your rice.

Location matters. Since rice grows in flooded fields, it can absorb a whole lot of arsenic. Rice from the southern United States, for example, tends to have more arsenic because of the insecticides used for years in the fields. Rice grown in Japan, on the other hand, often has less. Experts say to aim for rice from California, India, or Pakistan.

Arsenic tends to settle in the bran of rice, so brown rice holds on to about twice as much as white rice. To reduce exposure, wash your brown rice in water for a few minutes. Then cook it in excess water — at least 6 cups of water per cup of rice — and drain it once the grains are done. Limit brown rice to 3 cups or less each week by subbing a variety of whole grains into your menu.

Unprocessed perks — 3 unsung minerals take center stage

Brown rice is brimming with minerals that make it a nutritious choice for your meals. These three powerful nutrients top the charts, helping you hit your daily value.

Magnesium. Eating white rice isn't good enough if you want to meet your recommended amount of magnesium for the day. When brown rice is milled and polished to become white rice, it loses over 80% of its magnesium content. Having enough magnesium in your diet may help protect you from cardiovascular disease and diabetes. Fortunately, brown rice gives you 14% to 19% of your daily value in just 1 cup.

Selenium. A cup of brown rice contains about 27% of the amount of selenium you should be getting each day. That's good news because this trace element is vital to a properly working body. The mineral helps protect you from oxidative stress and infection, supports your thyroid, and even has a role in DNA production.

Manganese. This mineral often flies under the radar, but it's an essential part of many functions in your body. It plays a part in bone development and wound healing, just for starters. Plus brown rice is full of it. One cup of this food contains 77% to 98% of your recommended daily intake of manganese.

Oats

Feed on fiber to shrink belly fat faster

Oatmeal is a folksy cure for itchy skin. But if you want to tip the scale in your favor, don't bathe in it — eat it. Here's why.

The rising popularity of processed food means fiber-filled diets are falling by the wayside. Experts suspect that this change is a major player behind the growing rates of obesity. Oats could be part of the solution. And you have viscous soluble fiber to thank. It gels in your gut and slows down the digestion process. That means nutrients are absorbed more slowly, and you tend to feel fuller, longer.

This enduring satiety may in turn help with weight loss because you feel less hungry at your next meal. One astounding study even found that when eating the same number of calories at breakfast, participants who ate oatmeal stayed more full than those who had sugared cornflakes. In fact, by lunchtime, the people who ate the cornflakes were as hungry as those who drank only a glass of water for breakfast.

So is eating oats right when you wake up the smartest change you can make to your routine? Well, a research project studying effective weight loss techniques found that among folks who lost 30 pounds or more, and kept it off, more than 75% ate breakfast every morning. Other research suggests that people who regularly eat breakfast cereal, like oats or

Oats are great if you have celiac disease or a gluten intolerance because they're gluten free. But be wary of the cross-contamination that can happen during processing. Look for a gluten-free certified label to be safe.

porridge, have better overall diets and are more likely to get all the nutrients they need.

4 most common kinds of oats (and what to do with them)

The 18th-century English writer Samuel Johnson famously defined oats as "a grain, which in England is generally given to horses, but in Scotland supports the people." Joke's on him.

Oats have tons of nutritional value. And these days they come in different forms so you're bound to find an option that fits your needs, whether that means a leisurely breakfast ritual or a dash out the door. Here are four of the most common types you'll see at the store.

Steel-cut. When groats — whole oats with just the husk removed — are chopped up into a few pieces with steel blades, you get steel-cut oats. This process makes them nice and chewy but means they're not the best choice for baking recipes. They typically take about 20 to 30 minutes to cook on the stovetop, but they also prepare well in a slow cooker or pressure cooker.

Since steel-cut oats are less processed than rolled oats, they have slightly greater nutritional value. All oats are excellent for you, though. Just be cautious of added sugar, salt, or preservatives in whatever you choose.

Old-fashioned. If you have to pick just one type of oats, go with old-fashioned rolled oats. They are versatile and can be used in baked goods, granola bars, smoothies, and of course, as stovetop oatmeal.

Rolled oats are made by steaming the husked whole oat and rolling it between steam rollers. Because they're thinner, they only need about five to 10 minutes on your stove.

Quick-cooking. Another spin on rolled oats, quick oats are steamed and rolled. However, they're thinner than the old-fashioned style and may also be chopped into small pieces. This gives the oats a larger surface area, which cuts cooking time down to under five minutes. You can also substitute them into many recipes that call for rolled oats.

Instant. Need breakfast and need it now? Instant oats are your saving grace. All you have to do is pour in hot water, stir, and you're good to go in less than two minutes. That trim cooking time is possible because instant oats are typically precooked, dried, and chopped into small pieces after they've undergone the steaming and rolling process.

Instant oats should be left to porridge, though. Their super soft texture doesn't suit baked goods. Since they're the most processed type of oats, check their packaging for unnecessary additives.

 Kitchen hacks

Oats are an excellent food all on their own, but you can use them to enhance other dishes, too.

- Whether you eat them in a granola bar or as a breakfast cereal, oats have left their mark on morning meals. So why not add some to your breakfast smoothie? Pour in 1/4 cup of rolled oats per serving into your blender batch to make this tasty drink heartier.

- Help your budget go further by mixing oats into your ground beef. They can help bind the meat together like breadcrumbs if you're making meatballs or meatloaf, and you'll stretch out your beef supply. Combine a quarter cup of quick oats with each pound of beef before cooking.

- Blend rolled or quick oats into a fine powder. These ground oats work as a great flour alternative. Or use them to thicken your favorite soups, sauces, and dips.

Live longer when you lock out these big conditions

The one thing to eat more of to lower your chance of dying early from diabetes, heart disease, stroke, and cancer — whole grains. Shocked? A study of over 120,000 people revealed the link. Read on to find out why oats should be at the top of your list.

Drop your odds of diabetes by the spoonful. Cereal beta glucans are among the types of fiber most effective at preventing type 2 diabetes. And, you guessed it, oats are packed with them.

Beta glucan thickens the food in your digestive system, which slows the absorption of carbohydrates that are converted into glucose. This means glucose enters your bloodstream at a lower and slower rate. That leads to lower levels of insulin, the hormone responsible for helping glucose enter cells where it can be used for energy. Too much insulin can make your cells resistant to the hormone's effects, so this is good news all around.

Hang up on heart health hiccups. Across the globe, the No. 1 cause of death is cardiovascular disease. This includes conditions like heart disease and stroke. Fortunately, you can lower your risk through diet and lifestyle changes. One good option is adding oats into your meal plans. They contain heart-healthy fiber, iron, zinc, and magnesium, just for starters.

The nutrient doing most of the heavy lifting for your blood vessels is beta glucan fiber. It binds to bile acids that get excreted, causing your liver to pull from its cholesterol reserves to make more acids. That leads to less cholesterol in your bloodstream, where it could cause blockages.

To lower cholesterol, and therefore your risk of heart disease, experts recommend you get at least 3 grams of beta glucan each day. Some oat products offer that much in one to three servings.

Use oats to carve down your cancer risk. Research suggests that whole grains can reduce your chances of developing dangerous conditions like cancer. The dietary fiber and phenolic compounds in them may be behind this benefit.

- Both can improve your gut microbiome, which may affect how your body responds to cancer cells.

- Fiber works against various cancers in a number of ways. It might battle breast cancer, for example, by improving insulin resistance and lowering circulating estrogen levels.

- Phenolic compounds reduce oxidative damage to your cells and may alter how well cancer cells can spread.

Protect your eyesight with a bowl of this every day

That box of oats in your pantry has been eyeing you for weeks. Here's some good news that might finally convince you to crack it open. Feasting on oatmeal is a tasty way to reduce your risk of age-related macular degeneration (AMD).

This condition results from damage to the part of your eye called the macula, which controls sharp central vision. AMD is the leading cause of vision loss in people over the age of 65. Although it doesn't cause total blindness, you may have a harder time doing close-up tasks like cooking or home repairs. Driving, reading, and seeing faces may also prove more difficult.

Fortunately, when it comes to protecting your peepers, oatmeal pulls out all the stops. It has a low glycemic index, which means it won't raise your blood sugar levels quickly after you eat it. Research suggests that a low glycemic diet may help protect against early AMD and slow its progression into a more severe case. Experts theorize that this is because foods with a high glycemic index rapidly increase blood sugar to levels that cause cellular damage in your eyes.

Can't stand plain oatmeal? You can switch up the flavor and keep the glycemic index low by adding in some other flavor blasters that won't boost your blood sugar. Try tossing a few strawberries or pear slices on top alongside some chopped cashews.

 Bright idea

Take oats beyond the kitchen and target your rough, dry skin with a face mask. You can buy a pre-made mix from the store, or make your own.

Keep it simple with a basic recipe of blended oats and water, or add other nourishing ingredients like yogurt. Then head down to your toes for a foot soak. Add a few drops of essential oil to a tub of ground oats and warm water for a spa experience.

You can make a dry shampoo to spruce up your hair between washes, too. Massage a mix of equal parts ground oats and baking soda into your hair, wait a few minutes for the powder to absorb the oil, then brush it out.

Oats also help absorb oil from cooking or car maintenance mishaps. Sprinkle them over the spill and wait 10 minutes. Sweep up the mess and wipe away residue with a damp cloth.

Popcorn

Eat this fiber-filled snack for 2 belly benefits

You, like many other people, likely understand that fiber offers essential health benefits. Common ones include reducing the risk of obesity and improving digestion. You may also believe you're getting enough fiber. But that's often not the case. In fact, less than 10% of Americans are getting enough dietary fiber.

What can you do about this? Be sure to check the nutrition facts on all your packaged goods. The *American Journal of Lifestyle Medicine* recommends choosing foods with at least 3 grams of fiber per serving when possible. That's where popcorn comes in. A typical serving size is 3 cups and gives you about 3.5 grams of fiber for only 100 calories. Eureka!

All that fiber has amazing perks for your middle. Find out how it can ease some of your gut struggles.

Stay full with fiber. A large portion of your calories likely come from snacks. And it's easy to find yourself gorging on foods that lack nutrition between meals rather than fruits, veggies, and whole grains. Popcorn makes a great snack choice when you're trying to maintain or lose weight because of the fiber, which makes you feel fuller, and the low amount of calories.

Compare popcorn to chips, and you'll really see the benefits. Chips are a go-to savory snack in the U.S., but popcorn has a leg up in the health arena. Research shows that eating popcorn leaves you feeling less hungry than a similar calorie amount of chips, which could help you maintain a healthy weight.

Cut down constipation. When digested food moves through your colon too slowly, it hardens as the fluids are reabsorbed into your body. This makes stool difficult to pass. Insoluble fiber speeds up the movement of food in your digestive tract by pulling in water and adding bulk, which helps prevent and relieve constipation.

As a whole grain, popcorn is a good source of insoluble fiber. This is great for your body, and possibly your wallet, too. Some economic research suggests that over $12 billion spent in the U.S. on constipation-related health care costs could be saved if adults reached the recommended amount of fiber a day. That's 21 grams for women older than age 50 and 30 grams for men of the same age.

Unexpected ingredients puff up popcorn perks

"Popcorn may be the perfect snack food," says Joe Vinson, Ph.D., author of a study on surprising nutrients found in this crowd-pleaser. "It's the only snack that is 100% unprocessed whole grain."

For a long time, the benefits linked to whole grains — such as cancer and heart disease protection — were attributed to fiber. And although that's definitely an essential part, Vinson's research suggests there's another player at work, too. Polyphenols.

Corn isn't the only grain you can pop. Perk up amaranth, sorghum, quinoa, wheat berries, and more with the same simple skills you use to make popcorn. Many alternative grains stay small once popped, so they make excellent crunchy toppers on yogurt and salads, or mix them into homemade granola.

These compounds work as antioxidants. That means they guard you from dangerous molecules called free radicals that can damage the cells in your body. They're a key factor in why fruits and vegetables are leaders in reducing the risk of health-jeopardizing conditions. The same may hold true for whole grains, although they can't replace fresh produce in your diet.

Compared to other grains like oats, rice, and wheat, corn contains the highest amount of these antioxidants. That goes for the popcorn variety as well. And good news, experts also believe that popping it doesn't notably decrease the amount of antioxidants.

As such, popcorn's fiber paired with its polyphenols could make it the ultimate snack option. Just make sure your preparation method doesn't add buckets of salt and butter.

 Boost the benefits

Walking into a movie theater, you can't help but be drawn to that buttery popcorn aroma. Although enticing, this snack's benefits will be outweighed by the downsides of heavy salt and oil.

Keep popcorn's positives intact by staying old school and popping yours on the stove. Bonus — you'll get to pick your own serving size. Choose an oil that will give you a healthy portion of fat, like walnut or extra-virgin olive oil. Or skip oil entirely by air-popping the kernels. Then try one of these adventurous and nutritious toppings.

- Start simple and spritz your popcorn with balsamic vinegar. Then sprinkle on some chlorella, a nutrient-packed algae.

- Try a trail mix. Shake up a bag of popcorn with dried cranberries, your favorite chopped nuts, oats, and chocolate chips.

- Go for spice with chili lime. Toss your popcorn in a mixture of chili powder, ground cumin, lime zest, and salt. Finish with a squeeze of lime juice over top.

Quinoa

Pack a punch against chronic conditions with this pair of polyphenols

Quinoa, pronounced keen-wah, is a famous pseudo-cereal. That means it's not from the same plant family as grains, but it works undercover in your kitchen in similar ways as cereals like rice and barley. Unlike many other grains, though, quinoa is gluten free and it's a superior source of antioxidants.

These amazing substances neutralize free radicals in your body that could otherwise cause significant damage to your cells. Two key polyphenols in quinoa are kaempferol and quercetin. The antioxidant activity of these plant compounds helps keep you healthy. Find out how.

Stack up can-do kaempferol against cancer. Experts say kaempferol may reduce the risk of chronic diseases. In particular, studies show that eating more high-kaempferol foods is linked with lower cancer rates. Makes sense. The free radicals that antioxidants are so keen on defending against may play a role in cancer development.

But that's not all. Kaempferol's versatility enables it to attack cancer from multiple angles, which makes it such a great fighter. Test tube studies show that this polyphenol could also stop cancer cell growth and cause cancer cell death. Plus it may help protect your normal cells.

You can also find this powerful polyphenol in other foods like broccoli and beans, so make a night of it and prepare them in a dish with quinoa.

Quercetin quells dangerous conditions. Research suggests that among the flavonoids — a type of polyphenol — in quinoa, quercetin is the strongest antioxidant. Bad news for free radicals, but excellent news for you.

In its toolkit, quercetin also has anti-inflammatory and anti-histamine powers. What good are all these properties? Well, studies on quercetin suggest that it may protect against heart disease, cancer, and plaque buildup in your arteries.

Getting more quercetin-filled quinoa into your diet isn't as hard as you may think. Since it works in your kitchen like a grain, use it as one. Or to mix things up next time you bake a batch of bread, have a quarter of the flour come from quinoa. The flour is easy to make. Toast it in a skillet until lightly golden, then blend it into a powder.

 Boost the benefits

When it comes to cooking quinoa, the easiest way might actually be the best way. That's right, the health benefits of this food actually increase in the microwave.

Research has found that microwaving quinoa releases more phenolic acids and flavonoids than other cooking methods like roasting and boiling. You'll want to get in on the action since these polyphenols can help manage conditions like high blood sugar.

Making quinoa in the microwave takes less than 15 minutes. Start with 1 cup of freshly rinsed seeds in a microwave-safe bowl. Submerge them entirely in 2 cups of water, fully cover the bowl with a plate, and then place it in the microwave. Cook for six minutes, then let it rest for 30 seconds and give it a stir. Re-cover the bowl for another two minutes of cooking, then let it rest and absorb remaining liquid for another five minutes. Voila — 3 cups of steaming, scrumptious quinoa.

Fail-proof ways to prepare this colorful trio

Farmers around the world grow a combined 120 species of quinoa. But when you go shopping at the grocery store, the three main types you'll see are white, red, and black. You may also see "rainbow," but that isn't actually its own type. It's a tri-color mixture of the white, red, and black quinoa. Rather than the best of all worlds, this can make it a little difficult to cook.

If you want to give it a go, use it for porridge. Or keep them separate to make full use of their specialties. Here's a breakdown of these three types and their uses.

White. Among this trio, the one you're likely most familiar with is white quinoa. It has the largest seeds and softest texture. The flavor is slightly nutty. White quinoa is an easy substitute for rice, and its mild taste means it even works in baked goods. It has a cook time of just 10 to 15 minutes, although the age and amount of quinoa you're using will have an impact. Older quinoa may take longer and end up crunchier.

Wait! Before you start preparing your quinoa, be sure to rinse it off. This simple trick can help wash away the bitterness of quinoa's saponin coating. Saponins are anti-nutrients, which accounts for their undesirable flavor and means that they can reduce the absorption of nutrients like iron and magnesium.

Red. A strong nutty flavor and hearty crunch characterize red quinoa. You can use this type to replace rice or bulk up salads, but it doesn't mesh with sweet baked goods like the white variety. Red quinoa needs a few more minutes to cook than white. Between 15 and 20 minutes is typical.

Black. This type of quinoa has the thickest seed coating. The crunchier, sandy texture can make it a more daring choice. Its distinguishing texture and earthy but slightly sweet molasses flavor means it's best suited for recipes specifically designed with it in mind. Black quinoa takes the longest to cook at about 20 minutes.

Delicious milk stand-in helps you meet your protein goals

Getting enough protein in your diet without relying on meat doesn't have to be difficult. Quinoa is a plant food that's also a complete source of protein. That means it contains all nine essential amino acids, the building blocks of protein that your body can't make.

Proteins are the foundation of your body and make up your muscles, skin, organs, and beyond. The chains of amino acids that form proteins play a significant role in making hormones and brain chemicals, building muscle, and providing energy.

One cup of cooked quinoa has about 8 grams of protein. And if you often get your protein from dairy products like milk, you may be pleased to hear that you can actually make nutty, creamy quinoa milk at home. It's similar to oat milk and is an excellent use of cooked leftovers.

Leafy greens are an excellent source of nutrients, and quinoa greens are no exception. That includes quinoa leaves, sprouts, and microgreens — seedlings with baby leaves. Their healthful properties include being antimicrobial, antioxidant, and anti-cancer powerhouses. They're also a good source of essential minerals and amino acids.

All you need to do is blend 4 cups of water with 1 cup of cooked quinoa and a sweetener or flavoring, like vanilla extract or cinnamon. Strain the mixture, and store it in the fridge for up to four days.

You may want to skip using quinoa milk in hot drinks because it could curdle, but it makes a swell addition to baked goods, puddings, iced coffee, and more.

Crunch down on metabolic syndrome

Elevated blood pressure. High blood sugar. Abnormal cholesterol levels. Excess body fat around the waist. Each of them can be daunting alone, and when these conditions occur together they're called metabolic syndrome. They increase your risk of stroke, heart disease, obesity, and type 2 diabetes.

In the United States, metabolic syndrome is increasingly common. However, significant changes to your diet can help reduce your risk of developing more serious health conditions. Research suggests that adding quinoa to your meals is one such change that could make a difference.

That's because it can help reduce the level of a type of fat in your blood called triglycerides. You may have high triglycerides if you're regularly taking in more calories than you're burning off. Lowering triglyceride levels may decrease your odds of metabolic syndrome and reduce your risk of cardiovascular events.

In one study, overweight participants ate either 0, 25, or 50 grams of white quinoa seeds each day for three months. At the end of the study, the people who ate 50 grams — equal to about 3/4 cup of cooked quinoa — had lower triglyceride levels than they had at the start. Their levels were also lower than those who ate 25 grams a day or no quinoa.

Experts aren't certain why quinoa is so good at lowering triglyceride levels. Some theorize that the protein in it influences lipid absorption. Fiber also affects how much fat your small intestines take up, and at 5 grams per cup, quinoa is loaded with it.

Conquer poor nutrition with the mighty minerals of quinoa

There's more to quinoa than showstoppers like protein and antioxidants. This superfood is filled with minerals devoted to keeping your body in its best form. Here are a few you should know about, plus what percentage a cup of cooked quinoa contributes toward reaching the recommended amount, or daily value (DV).

- **51% to 65% DV of manganese.** Quinoa is rich in this element that's essential to a functioning metabolism. The trace mineral also assists enzymes, which speed along chemical reactions in your body.

- **40% DV of phosphorus.** Fun fact, phosphorus is the second most-abundant mineral in your body and makes up approximately 1% of your total body weight. Its main role is forming your bones and teeth. But it also works alongside B vitamins for kidney function, muscle contractions, and more.

- **39% DV of copper.** This mineral helps your body absorb iron, and the two work together to form red blood cells. Copper is also key to keeping your nerves and bones healthy. Your body can't make its own, so you have to get copper from food.

- **35% DV of iron.** Known for its essential role in hemoglobin, iron helps carry oxygen through your body. It also helps maintain healthy connective tissue.

- **28% to 37% DV of magnesium.** Low of levels of magnesium may be connected to health risks like high blood pressure and cardiovascular disease. Fortunately, 1 cup of quinoa can give you about 118 milligrams of magnesium.

A closer look
Ancient grains

They're the oldest new trend on grocery shelves and in online shopping carts — ancient grains. These pseudo-cereals and grains, by definition, have remained largely unaltered over the last thousand years. Many of them have more minerals, fiber, and protein than modern, genetically modified whole grains like rice and corn.

You're probably already seeing ancient grains as ingredients in processed foods like breads, crackers, and breakfast cereals. The whole and flour versions are popping up on shelves, too, though they can be harder to find in stores and are often more expensive than their modern counterparts.

That said, this is one bandwagon you might want to hop on. Along with crowd favorites like barley, sorghum, and quinoa, take these up-and-coming options for a test drive.

Amaranth. Called the "food of immortality" by the Aztecs, this gluten-free ancient grain is actually a seed. It has a crunchy texture similar to quinoa, and its nutty, herbal taste complements sweet muffins as well as savory soups. It also works well in place of couscous, rice, oatmeal, and pasta.

A cup of cooked amaranth will serve up 65% of your daily recommended iron. That's five times more iron than you'll find in wheat.

Bon appétit — you'll want to eat up the whole grains within four months if you keep them in your panty, or eight months if stored in the freezer.

Farro. Nutty and chewy, farro is a great stand-in for barley. But wait, three types of ancient grains are often marketed as farro, so it's up to you to scan the package for clues.

- Farro piccolo (*Triticum monococcum*), known as einkorn, is the smallest of the three.

- Farro medio (*Triticum dicoccum*) is most common in the U.S. and is often called emmer.

- Farro grande (*Triticum spelta*), or spelt, has 25% to 36% of the fiber you need each day in 1 cup of the cooked grain.

Pearled and semi-pearled farro cooks faster, between 15 and 30 minutes. Whole farro, which has all of the nutritious bran intact, will take longer and requires a soak beforehand. Grain lovers agree, it's worth the wait.

Khorasan wheat. This buttery-tasting grain is known most commonly under the brand name KAMUT. Trademarked by farmers Mack and Bob Quinn in 1990, the name means it's been grown organically and hasn't been hybridized or modified.

"More people are learning about ancient grains and their myriad health benefits, and are looking for new ways to incorporate these superfoods into their diet," says Bob Quinn. "While ancient grains, like KAMUT wheat, are already included in many products on the market, such as pasta, cereal, and granola, they can also be easily swapped with regular wheat to make your favorite recipes more delicious and nutritious."

You can also use it in place of rice in pilaf and casserole recipes. A smart move since a cup of cooked KAMUT has 9.8 grams of protein — double the amount you'd get in a cup of cooked brown rice.

Teff. It's the world's smallest grain, but it makes up for it in a big way. In fact, these poppy-sized seeds have more calcium than many other grains, with 10% to 12% of the amount seniors need each day in every cup of cooked teff.

Teff flour is famous as the main ingredient in injera. But if you're not up for making this Ethiopian flatbread, you can sub it into your own favorite baked goods, including pancakes and breads. Replace up to a fourth of the flour in your recipe with teff flour to add nutrition and flavor.

Because they're so small, the gluten-free whole grains cook in 15 to 20 minutes. Perfect for adding a last-minute exotic flare to stews, salads, and veggie burgers.

If you can't find teff in your local supermarket, alongside other whole grains or in the baking or breakfast aisle, you can always look for it online.

Sorghum

Go with the grain for a healthier heart

The United States is the world's leading producer of the nutrient-rich grain sorghum. Yet, it's used most frequently as animal feed or a fuel alternative. A growing reputation for its health benefits, though, could change that. Get ahead of the curve by adding sorghum to your diet, and make your heart happy.

Fantastic surprise from these fats. Two of the most common types of fatty acids in the white, red, and black varieties of sorghum are oleic and linoleic acid. These are both healthy unsaturated fats.

How good for you are they? Well, they may reduce the risk of thrombosis, which is when blood clots block veins or arteries. That's because they help keep fats and cholesterol from accumulating in your arteries, causing them to narrow. Called atherosclerosis, this buildup can block blood flow and may lead to a blood clot.

Two types of nutrients tame your ticker. Sorghum is simply full of minerals and antioxidants, and some of them have been identified as potential heart healers.

- For instance, sorghum contains both potassium and sodium. Having a balanced ratio of these minerals could help protect against chronic conditions like high blood pressure and stroke.

- Antioxidants, including polyphenols and carotenoids, are particularly plentiful in the outer bran layer of sorghum grains. Experts recommend eating foods rich in antioxidants as one method of preventing heart disease.

Watch out

Sorghum is safe for those with gluten allergies, but that doesn't necessarily mean it's safe for everyone to eat. That's because sorghum is a grass, and many people have allergic reactions to grasses or grass pollen.

Stop eating sorghum if you experience any food allergy symptoms like tingling, itching, or swelling in or around your mouth. Other severe symptoms include abdominal pain, nausea, fainting, or even anaphylaxis.

Get the basics down: Storing and preparing sorghum

The type of sorghum you're most likely to find at grocery stores comes from the plant called grain sorghum. But don't assume every option on the shelf is a whole grain with all parts intact. Read the label. The pearled variety has the nutritious bran removed, while the flour may be made from either whole or refined grains.

The flour has been described as the gluten-free alternative that's most similar to standard wheat flour. But if you have a severe sensitivity, like celiac disease, check the label to make sure your sorghum products were made in a gluten-free facility.

Even if you don't need to exclude gluten from your diet, you'll want to add this ancient grain into your meal planning. Besides being milled into flour, this grain is great popped, flattened into cereal-like flakes, or boiled. Those options get you a heaping dose of nutrients like magnesium, potassium, and B vitamins.

Sorghum has a mild flavor that includes a slight nutty sweetness with an undercurrent of earthiness. It has a firm texture, and when you chew sorghum spheres you may feel them "pop" in your mouth.

Sorghum takes a little longer than many other grains to cook, so give yourself more time to get it ready. Prepare it on your stovetop in a large pot with 1 cup of sorghum to 3 cups of liquid, like water or broth, along with a pinch of salt. Bring it to a boil, and leave it covered while it simmers for 45 to 60 minutes. Afterward, let it stand for five minutes, then fluff with a fork and serve.

Cooked sorghum pairs well with veggies such as mushrooms, eggplants, and roasted carrots. Some delicious add-ins include lemon juice, garlic, lentils, lime, and ginger. Or sweeten it up with ingredients like coconut milk, cinnamon, and raisins.

If you have leftover uncooked sorghum grains, store them in a sealed container. As long as moisture is kept out, it can last about four months. Cooked sorghum will stay fresh in a refrigerated, sealed container for a few days.

A simple swap to mill down sugar spikes

Millets are small-seeded grasses that double as defeaters of diabetes. That's because this type of food, which includes sorghum, has a low glycemic index (GI).

The glycemic index ranks foods on a scale from 0 to 100. A bigger score means a food spikes blood sugar levels higher and faster after a meal than a lower score would. Sorghum's glycemic index varies slightly between types, like whole grain versus flour, but generally falls in the 60s.

That's notably lower than common grains like white rice, with a GI of 71.7, and refined wheat, with a GI of 74.2. Western diets tend to emphasize processed grains like these, so swapping some out for the underutilized millets may be beneficial in the prevention and management of type 2 diabetes.

A recent paper suggests that the difference in GI score is what makes the millet types they studied, which averaged a GI of 52.7, so promising. This study, published in *Frontiers in Nutrition*, found that regularly eating millets reduced average post-meal blood sugar levels by about 15% in people with diabetes.

The researchers also took a look at HbA1c levels — average blood sugar levels over the past three months — which is a measure of long-term glycemic control. They found that participants with diabetes and pre-diabetes who ate millets for three months or longer had lower HbA1c levels than those whose diets were centered around rice and wheat.

This benefit likely stems in part from millets' high fiber content. The key is making them a regular part of your meal plans.

 Kitchen hacks

Legend has it that doctors once prescribed a tablespoon of sorghum syrup daily to help people get more iron, calcium, and potassium in the times before multivitamins. Now it makes a great swap for molasses.

Both molasses and sorghum syrup are dark brown with a thick consistency. However, molasses comes from sugar cane whereas sorghum syrup, also called sorghum molasses, comes from the stalks of the plant known as sweet sorghum.

In recipes asking for molasses, you can sub in sorghum syrup in a 1-to-1 ratio. Sorghum syrup is lower in total sugar than molasses but is sweeter, so you may want to consider using less. It also works well in marinades and dressings.

If you can't find this sweetener on your supermarket shelves, look for it online. When picking yours out, check the label to see if it's 100% sorghum syrup. Some products may be diluted with unhealthy corn syrup. Store it like honey in a cool, dark place in a jar with a tight-fitting lid.

Wheat bran

4 reasons your gut will thank you for eating more of this

Eat this kind of cereal daily, and help prevent hemorrhoids, constipation, colon cancer, and even weight gain. It's high-fiber bran to the rescue. Not just any kind of fiber will do. That's because the different types have different effects. But wheat bran offers insoluble fiber that could be invaluable.

Hold off hemorrhoids. In the U.S., 1 in 20 people experience hemorrhoids. These inflamed, swollen veins occur around the anus or in the lower rectum and can cause pain, irritation, and even bleeding. Eating high-fiber foods is one of the best ways to prevent hemorrhoids. Fiber increases stool weight and water retention, which allows stool to pass more quickly with less strain.

Fiber counteracts constipation. The stool-softening quality of insoluble fibers like wheat bran is also what makes them useful against constipation. Just be sure to choose coarse wheat bran. Research shows this type will increase stool water content, which has the softening effect, but finely ground wheat bran decreases water content and has the opposite effect.

Reduce your risk of colorectal cancer. Colorectal cancer is one of the most common kinds of cancer in the world, and it is second only to lung cancer in the leading causes of cancer death. However, some data suggests that over 40% of cases could be prevented with lifestyle changes. One route is to improve your eating and drinking habits. High-fiber foods in particular may have a protective effect. A possible reason for this is that an increase in stool bulk dilutes carcinogens, lessening exposure in your intestines.

This food won't weigh you down. Bumping up your daily fiber intake could help you hold off weight gain. That's because one major contributing factor to obesity is taking in more energy from your food than you're using up.

Getting more fiber keeps you feeling full and your nutrient levels high while lowering energy absorption. Insoluble fiber may be especially helpful for losing weight if you're eating high amounts of fat.

Bran wars: Wheat beats oat for certain concerns

Bran is the hard outer layer of cereal grains, whether you're talking wheat or oat. And it's heralded by nutritionists and chefs alike.

Some things hold true across these different types of bran. For instance, wheat and oat bran both make excellent additions to baked goods and should be stored in a cool, dark place, like a sealed container in your pantry or fridge. These two also provide a variety of vitamins and minerals, like magnesium and thiamine, for hearty health benefits.

One key difference between them is that oats are naturally gluten-free and wheat bran is not. Another notable distinction is that although they're both great sources of fiber, wheat bran offers insoluble fiber and oat bran mainly contains soluble fiber.

This makes wheat bran a slightly better option for keeping your digestion regular. Oat bran on the other hand might help with lowering cholesterol.

Whip up your new favorite breakfast for better blood pressure

Start your morning stress-free with a meal that offers a surplus of benefits. Wheat bran is an excellent source of fiber, roughage that's great not only for your digestion but for your blood pressure (BP). That's right, some research suggests that dietary fiber can reduce the risk of hypertension.

Get your BP readings off to a good start first thing each day. Wheat bran is highly versatile in the field of morning meals, and that means you have a ton of great options.

> The rough texture of wheat bran makes it useful as a skin exfoliant, and turning it into a body scrub is simple. Just mix 2 tablespoons of wheat bran, 1 teaspoon of baking soda, and 1 teaspoon of coconut oil together in a bowl. Smooth it out with a little bit of water, gently scrub, then rinse it off.

- Make your own bran flakes with an online recipe, or simplify things and buy bran flakes already made — just watch out for added sugar. Toss some sliced banana on the side for extra flavor and fiber.

- Not only is wheat bran an excellent addition to baked goods, but you can replace some of the flour in those recipes with it. Whip it up in some muffins, banana bread, pancakes, or waffles.

- Need something simpler at 6 a.m.? Try sprinkling wheat bran on top of your favorite smoothie, yogurt, or cold and hot cereals for a fiber fill-up.

Getting more fiber is all well and good, but take it slowly. Adding too much wheat bran to your diet all at once can cause tummy troubles like bloating and gas. You can help ward off these side effects by increasing your fluids, too, in order to keep all that fiber moving along in your pipes.

A closer look
Best breads

It's like a game show. Rows and rows of bread, and you have to pick the healthiest. Quick. You scan the package for a "made with wheat" statement or a "good source of fiber" claim. Bad move. Avoid these top mistakes folks make when shopping for bread if you want to win this round.

Assuming "wheat" means healthy. "Wheat" tells you what type of grain is in the bread, but if you're looking for more whole grains you need more details. The first ingredient should be "100% whole wheat" or "100% whole grain," which means the grains are not refined.

Not understanding "multigrain." The word simply means it's made of more than one type of grain. Those grains could be refined, so check out the ingredients list.

Neglecting the fiber rule. According to experts at Harvard, you should make sure whole-grain foods contain at least 1 gram of fiber per 10 grams of total carbohydrates. The simplest way to do this is divide the amount of carbs by 10. The amount of fiber in the bread should be at least as high as the result.

Overlooking other ingredients. First check the serving size. Some breads are listed as one slice, but how often do you eat a one-slice sandwich? Then skim the label for salt and sweeteners like honey, corn syrup, and cane juice. Stick to an option with less than 2 grams of sugar and less than 150 milligrams of salt per slice.

Shopping by color. Whole-wheat bread is often darker, but that doesn't mean darker breads are always healthier. Food companies may pull a fast one and dye their bread brown. Don't fall for it.

Only browsing the bread aisle. Breads without preservatives go bad faster. The solution? Store them in the freezer. So why aren't you perusing the freezer section for better breads, including whole-grain sprouted options?

And, of course, you wouldn't want to neglect your local in-store bakery. You may find healthier, freshly baked breads with fewer, but higher quality, ingredients.

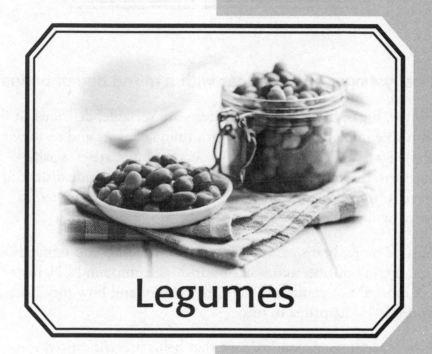

Legumes

Beans

Feel younger and stronger with a mixed bag of beans

Pintos, limas, black-eyed peas. Beans are versatile, delicious, and available in many varieties, all with unique flavors and textures to delight your palate. They're perfect in soups, stews, salads, burritos, casseroles, and cooked on their own as a side dish. You have so many ways to prepare and flavor them, it's easy to eat some with every meal.

What's more, beans contain at least five vitamins and minerals and are full of fiber and other nourishing compounds. Here's a bit more about common nutrients in beans and how they help you stay in the prime of life.

- Vitamin E. An antioxidant that helps prevent cancer, this vitamin boosts your immune system and blocks clots from forming in your arteries.

- B vitamins. Help your body break down food into energy. Beans are high in B6, which may combat cancer, especially in the colon.

- Selenium. Another cancer fighter that helps protect against cell damage and infections.

- Manganese. This mineral is absolutely vital for your brain and nerve function.

- Potassium. Helps lower blood pressure and reduce your risk of cardiovascular disease.

- Fiber. Keeps you full, may bind and remove toxins from your body through digestion, and helps regulate blood sugar levels. Beans are one of the top fiber sources you can get in your diet, including white beans, navy beans, and adzuki beans.

Antioxidant-rich beans, a key factor in anti-aging. Oxidative stress — this damage happens when rogue molecules wreak havoc on your cells. Many experts believe that an accumulation of that cell damage contributes to aging as well as conditions like diabetes, cancer, obesity, and heart disease.

But beans have a secret weapon. Polyphenols. These special plant compounds act as antioxidants to neutralize dangerous molecules that cause oxidative stress. Common varieties like kidney beans, black beans, and pinto beans don't seem so ho-hum after all.

The secret to remaining hale and hearty for life. As you get older, your muscles grow weaker. And sarcopenia, age-related muscle loss, can make you prone to injuries and falls. But keep active and include beans at every meal, and your muscles can stay nice and healthy. Beans contain one nutrient your body must have to stay strong as you age — protein. It helps repair, build, and preserve muscle, keeping you stable and injury-free.

> Dry beans are much cheaper than canned versions and lower in sodium. Wondering how many dry beans you need to make a recipe using canned or already-cooked beans? For every 1 cup of dry beans, you'll end up with 2 to 2 1/2 cups of cooked beans.

You should aim to get at least 0.36 grams of protein per pound of body weight each day for the best benefits. Simply multiply your weight by 0.36 to figure out what's right for your body. Fortunately, beans are the perfect solution for getting enough muscle-saving protein. Load up on cranberry beans, split peas, and more to maintain muscle and remain mobile.

Boost the benefits

Dry beans are money-saving and convenient to store in your pantry for nutritious fiber and protein-packed meals. But even though you can keep them long term, they need proper storage in order to stay fresh and tasty.

Keep your dry beans in airtight containers such as sealed bags or glass jars. Vacuum-sealed bags or containers may provide additional benefits, such as preserving freshness longer and eliminating any potential insects. Store your packed beans out of light in a cool environment. If you choose bags for storage, place them inside a hard, sealed container to protect from bugs and rodents.

You can store beans indefinitely, but use them within one to three years for the best flavor. If you've had your beans for longer than one year or if they aren't as fresh as you'd like, try adding a pinch of baking soda while cooking to soften tough beans.

Eat the rainbow for more fiber and better health

Noshing on the same type of bean week after week — boring! Why stick to one when you can sample from a rainbow of options? Feast your eyes on white, red, green, black, and even speckled beans. Adding these to your plate provides variety and helps you fill up on fiber — a health powerhouse.

A cup of cooked white navy beans, for instance, provides 64% to 91% of the amount of fiber you need each day. Red adzuki beans are close behind with 56% to 80% of your daily value per cooked cup. Green mung beans ring in at 51% to 73% per cooked cup.

Whichever type of bean you choose, here's why eating plenty of fiber is incredibly beneficial.

- helps you feel full, so you can maintain a healthy weight

- improves digestion, keeping bowel movements regular

- is associated with a decreased risk of colorectal and breast cancer

- lowers "bad" LDL cholesterol levels and your odds of heart disease

- balances blood sugar, lowering your chances of developing type 2 diabetes

- reduces risk of diverticulosis, which happens when small pouches bulge from the digestive tract

✗ Kitchen hacks

The secret to faster-cooking beans is a good soak. To get started, discard wrinkly or strange beans and debris. Then use one of these three soaking methods.

- **Hot soaking makes cooking quicker and reduces gas.** Place your beans in a pot and cover with water — 10 cups of water for 2 cups of beans. Bring to a boil for three minutes, remove from heat, and let stand covered for four hours.

- **Traditional soaking is best for pressure cooking or planning ahead.** Set your beans in a pot with cold water for eight hours or overnight.

- **Try quick soaking for fast beans.** Cover beans with water in a pot — 6 cups of water for 2 cups of beans. Bring to a boil for two to three minutes. Remove from heat and cover for one hour.

After the soak, drain and rinse. To cook on a stove, simmer covered in water until tender, 30 minutes to two hours. Now your beans are ready for your favorite recipes.

A 'Great' way to beat metabolic syndrome

Metabolic syndrome is a group of conditions that include obesity, high cholesterol, elevated blood pressure, and high blood sugar. Having this syndrome increases your chances of developing type 2 diabetes and cardiovascular disease.

One of the best ways to tackle metabolic syndrome, and stay off prescriptions, is to improve your diet. That's where this one phenomenal food comes in — Great Northern beans. Eat more of these to reduce heart disease, blood sugar, and weight.

Protect your ticker from heart disease and stroke. Eating lots of beans is associated with a lower risk of heart disease. And no wonder. A study published in *The Journal of Nutrition* links having lower blood pressure with getting more protein from plant sources.

"High blood pressure is one of the most potent risk factors for developing cardiovascular disease," says lead researcher Amy Jennings, Ph.D. "A reduction in blood pressure leads to a reduction in mortality caused by stroke or coronary heart disease." And she says that changing your diet to include more beans and other sources of protein could help.

Doubling up on stroke protection, beans also supply vitamin B6 and magnesium, which are both linked to a lower risk of brain attacks. Vitamin B6 helps break down homocysteine — an amino acid that can increase stroke risk if not properly broken down. Researchers think the protective effect of magnesium may be related to lowering blood pressure. As luck would have it, a cup of canned Great Northern beans contains 16% to 19% of the B6 you need each day, and 32% to 42% of your daily magnesium.

Combat type 2 diabetes with beans. Putting beans on your plate can help you balance blood sugar, which may ward off type 2 diabetes. And Great Northern beans are perfect for the job. Like other beans, they're low on the glycemic index, which rates foods based on how much they spike your blood sugar. Adding these white beans to your diet in place of processed meats and refined carbs like white rice may be the most delicious way to keep your blood sugar stable.

Whittle your waistline with fiber and protein. Preventing metabolic syndrome typically requires weight loss. But the bad news is that most people who lose weight see the pounds return over time. Finding foods that satisfy you and keep you full — in other words, have plenty of fiber and protein — is the secret to lasting weight loss.

Research shows that people who eat beans regularly have lower body weight, smaller waists, and less chance of becoming overweight or obese. That 13 grams of fiber and 19 grams of protein found in a cup of canned Great Northern beans isn't going to waste — or your waist.

A heartwarming gift that's easy on your wallet

Soup In a Jar is often called Friendship Bean Soup, and for a good reason. You'll make fast friends with this healthy, edible gift. What's more, it's simple to assemble and delicious. Gather a wide-mouth quart-sized jar with a lid, a small zip-top baggie, label, and these ingredients.

- 3/4 cup each of five types of beans of your choice
- 2 tablespoons each of bouillon granules, dried onion flakes, dried basil, and dried parsley
- 1 teaspoon each of paprika, dry mustard, rosemary, garlic powder, oregano, and salt

Add beans to the jar in layers. Pour seasonings into the baggie and place on top of beans. Seal the jar, and add a label with these instructions.

- Rinse beans and place in a large pot. Cover with water.
- Bring to a boil, then cover and let rest for an hour.
- Rinse beans and add back to the pot along with the seasoning mix, a 14-ounce can of diced tomatoes, and 6 cups of water.
- Let simmer for about two hours, until beans are tender. Makes 12 servings.

A closer look
Bean swaps

Give your budget a break and sub out pricey meats for beans. The Academy of Nutrition and Dietetics says it's a top way to slash spending on groceries. More than a big money saver, though, beans are a scrumptious and nutritious stand-in for all sorts of fare.

adzuki beans	Also called red beans, don't confuse adzukis with kidney beans. Adzukis are smaller and have a nutty, sweet taste that makes them popular in desserts. Puree cooked adzukis and mix into your brownie recipe instead of flour and sugar.
black beans	The mild, creamy flavor of black beans pairs well with spicy burritos and enchiladas. For a new twist, replace starchy veggies like whipped potatoes with a black bean mash.
cannellini beans	Nutty cannellini beans may be a favorite in soups, pastas, and salads, but replace 1/2 or all the ricotta cheese in your lasagna recipe with pureed cannellinis and you'll really amp up the nutrition.
chickpeas	Coarsely mashed chickpeas have a flavor and texture that can mimic chicken or turkey, making them a delicious swap for poultry in salads.
Great Northern beans	Replace 1/2 or all the butter in your banana bread recipe with a batch of pureed Great Northern beans. No one will ever know the difference.
kidney beans	For healthier nachos, forget about ground meat and top crispy tortilla chips with kidney beans. Finish with reduced-fat cheese, nonfat Greek yogurt, salsa, and some fresh scallions.
lentils	Substitute 1 pound of ground meat with 2 cups of cooked, drained lentils the next time sloppy Joes are on your menu. The meaty, earthy flavor will have guests dishing up seconds. Precooked boxed or canned lentils will work when time is short.
lima beans	Say bye-bye to bacon's unhealthy fat and calories. Toss 1 1/2 cups of cooked lima beans with 1 tablespoon of chili powder, smoked paprika, or your favorite spice blend. Roast at 400 degrees for about 40 minutes or until lightly browned. Then sprinkle these crispy lima snacks anywhere you'd use bacon bits.
navy beans	Puree cooked navy beans until smooth and creamy, then season to your taste. Serve as a healthy mayonnaise alternative on sandwiches or use as a dip for fresh veggies.
pinto beans	Pinto beans may be a speckled brown color, but they taste similar to black beans. Mash pintos until chunky and replace 1/2 or all the ground beef in your next burger.

Chickpeas

Powerhouse pulse: Don't miss out on these fantastic nutrients

Chickpeas have long been a key part of Mediterranean and Middle Eastern cuisine. It's easy to see why. This mildly nutty-flavored legume is eaten cold in salads, hot in stews, and roasted in crunchy snacks. Let's not even get into the wonders of homemade hummus.

As if that's not enough, chickpeas also pack a powerful nutritional punch. They're an excellent source of protein and fiber, and contain copious amounts of vitamins to help you stay healthy as you age.

> Green chickpeas are a younger variety, harvested in late spring to early summer before becoming fully ripened and dried. They have a creamy texture, almost buttery, with a flavor like spring peas. You can snack on them right out of the pod, place them in a salad, or steam and serve like edamame.

Tap into the benefits of vitamin B6. While the English-speaking world prefers the word "chickpea," Spanish speakers are partial to "garbanzo." Either way, this legume has lots of vitamin B6 to keep your nervous and immune systems running smoothly. In fact, just 1 cup of canned chickpeas provides older folks with more than half the amount they need each day.

Here's another reason you'll want to load up. A recent European study found that seniors who got more vitamin B6 in their diets took less time getting out of a chair. No wonder, since this vitamin is needed for proper muscle function. And among those seniors who didn't exercise much, high levels of this nutrient were associated with a greater ability to grip things. That's a skill you need to carry groceries, for example, or turn a doorknob.

Don't forget that folate is your friend. This vitamin is necessary for healthy red blood cell formation, as well as cell growth. And some research suggests that it might be helpful in treating depression.

Animal studies suggest that folate may also be connected to living longer. While researchers aren't yet ready to champion this vitamin as the next fountain of youth, it can't hurt to munch on some chickpeas while you wait for the data to come in.

Hard to believe, but this little legume contains three times more folate per serving than the popular "king" of greens, kale. In fact, a cup of canned chickpeas provides 161 micrograms of this vitamin. That's 40% of your daily needs. Just be sure to rinse them in cold water before eating. Doing so reduces the salt content and makes for easier digestion.

Easy-to-make roasted super snack

Leblebi is a roasted chickpea snack popular in Turkey. They have the right idea. Some research shows that leblebi has more resistant starch than raw chickpeas.

Resistant starch is like fiber, going right to your colon undigested. There, it feeds friendly bacteria and increases certain fatty acids, which could have a ton of good-for-you side effects. That includes improving digestion, balancing blood sugar, and lowering appetite.

Want to get in on the action? Make your own roasted chickpeas at home. Many recipes are available, whether you use canned chickpeas or dry chickpeas, soaked overnight. Also, you can use many different seasoning blends, from garlic-onion to ranch powder.

Preheat the oven to 400 degrees. Strain and rinse your chickpeas, and blot them dry with paper towels. Toss with olive oil and season to taste. Spread the beans on a cookie sheet and bake 35 to 45 minutes, until crunchy.

Hummus: A nutritional powerhouse

Is it possible to find a snack that contains a wealth of super-foods? That's hummus.

The main ingredient is pureed chickpeas. After all, hummus means "chickpea" in Arabic. Chickpeas contain protein and fiber, plus manganese, copper, folate, magnesium, and much more.

Hummus has existed for so many centuries, its country of origin is unknown. Today, it's popular in many areas around the world, and has enjoyed growing popularity in the U.S.

Recipes traditionally combine chickpeas with garlic, tahini, lemon juice, salt, and olive oil. With all its healthy ingredients, hummus is much more nutritious than typical snack food.

Commercial versus homemade hummus. You can't beat the convenience of store-bought hummus, and so many varieties. However, homemade is not difficult to make, and it's you who's in control. For example, you can puree chickpeas while still warm for a smoother, creamier result. Also, you can make it according to your taste, and drop ingredients you don't want such as soybean oil, citric acid, and potassium sorbate.

> For added flavor, enjoy some hummus varieties — whether bought or homemade. The possibilities are endless, from garlic, jalapeno, red pepper, and cilantro to black bean, spinach, and Mediterranean style. You can even go sweet with dark chocolate. Let your palate be your guide, but remember to keep all your add-ins healthy.

Regardless of which kind you choose, follow this advice.

- Watch the sodium. In many commercial varieties, you might find up to 200 milligrams in just 2 tablespoons. So be sure to review the nutrition label.

- Watch your portions. You could get carried away and dip too much. Keep in mind that one serving is just 2 level tablespoons.

Hummus is far more than a dip. There's no shortage of ways to add hummus to your diet. Here are several ideas.

- Make a chicken and hummus brown rice casserole.
- Add it to a rotini pasta salad.
- Make it a pizza topping.
- Create a condiment, replacing mayo or mustard.
- Add it to a vegan wrap.
- Put it in mashed potatoes instead of sour cream.
- Turn it into a sauce with sesame oil, and toss it with spaghetti noodles.

It's aquafabulous — tap into the delicious magic of bean water and other kitchen scraps

Stop! Are you throwing out the liquid from that can of tasty chickpeas? What you might see as destined for the drain is actually an egg white substitute that's truly revolutionary for vegans, those suffering from egg allergies, or anyone looking to make the most of their grocery store dollars.

Called aquafaba, this syrupy bean water is a mix of proteins, starches, and minerals released from the chickpeas during cooking. You can use it straight from the can to thicken, bind, or blend ingredients in many recipes, like homemade mayo. Three tablespoons of aquafaba equals one egg. But the true magic happens when you whip it.

Experts say you'll get stiff but fluffy results by whipping aquafaba with a bit of cream of tartar — 1/4 teaspoon to 4 ounces of aquafaba. Then use this light foam to make meringues, or fold into your favorite muffin, cake, or bread recipe.

But don't stop this reclaiming kick you're on. Look around the kitchen for other items nearly everyone tosses out — but shouldn't. You'll find plenty of useful kitchen scraps just begging to be salvaged.

- When the last pickle is gone, drop your own fresh veggies into the brine for homemade relish.

- Toss clean potato peels with olive oil and seasonings, then roast in the oven for a crunchy snack.

- Simmer scraped corn cobs with some herbs, then use the stock for chowder or when cooking grains.

- Slightly bruised fruit is still yummy when turned into a smoothie or jam.

- Orange, lime, or lemon peels absorb cooking odors when simmered with water, cinnamon sticks, and whole cloves.

- Stale bread is perfect for croutons or breadcrumbs.

- Save the stems from herbs like basil, cilantro, and parsley, and let them flavor stock, dressings, pesto, or stuffing.

 Bright idea

Whole chickpeas are tasty in pastas, sandwich spreads, soups, and curries. But don't cork your creativity. Have fun with these surprising chickpea products.

- Chickpea flour. Simply grind dry chickpeas into powder, and you have chickpea flour. Also known as gram flour or besan, it's a staple in India and used throughout the world. Chickpea flour is a healthy, gluten-free addition to many dishes, loaded with vitamins, minerals, protein, and fiber. Use it as an egg substitute due to its binding properties, a soup and sauce thickener, or whole wheat flour substitute.

- Chickpea coffee. Get your own nutritional, caffeine-free coffee fix like many have done for centuries. To make your own, roast the chickpeas at 300 degrees on a cookie sheet until they look like roasted coffee beans. Grind in a blender or coffee grinder, keeping in mind that bigger chunks leave less residue when brewing. Boil, strain, and serve.

Lentils

Eating for iron — nature's way to a healthier you

Your parents weren't kidding when they encouraged you to eat healthy foods. After all, that's the best way to get your vitamins and minerals. And lentils are one of the most nourishing things you can eat.

These tiny, lens-shaped legumes are packed with iron. Your bone marrow needs this mineral to produce hemoglobin, a protein that enables red blood cells to carry oxygen throughout your body. Without enough iron, you may feel tired, weak, and dizzy.

But back to the mighty lentil. Just 1 cup of this cooked legume has a whopping 6.6 milligrams of iron. That's 83% of your recommended daily amount. So eat more lentils — they'll also help you avoid the following health issues.

Put restless legs syndrome (RLS) to rest. Anyone with RLS is familiar with the uncomfortable leg sensations that cause an overwhelming urge to get up and move. Symptoms are often worse at night, and can range from aching to itching.

Researchers believe RLS likely arises from low iron levels in the brain. That's where lentils come in. Along with all that iron, they contain lots of folate and magnesium — two nutrients that have been shown to ease the symptoms of RLS.

Lentils can help your ticker. Did you know that people with heart failure often have an iron deficiency? It's true. The cells responsible for your heart's rhythmic beating depend on this mineral to function properly.

But here's the neat part. When you're eating lentils for their iron, you'll also get special compounds called polyphenols. Studies have found that these micronutrients, along with other substances in lentils, are connected to lower rates of cardiovascular disease. So start cooking!

Boost your immune system with iron. Of course, proper diet and nutrition are key to remaining healthy. And iron is an essential part of that. It plays a vital role in your immune response, your first line of defense against disease and infections.

You'll also want to know that people with long-term iron deficiencies produce fewer and fewer antibodies. Those are your immune system's search-and-destroy army of blood proteins that hunt down and neutralize foreign invaders like fungi and parasites. More lentils anyone?

Thinning hair may not be hopeless. Most doctors don't realize there's a link between iron deficiency and hair loss. But that's what 40 years of research shows, according to Cleveland Clinic dermatologists. One possible reason? Iron is an essential component of an enzyme that assists in hair growth.

It makes sense, then, that thinning hair could mean you need more of this nutrient. The best way to get it is through eating more iron-rich foods like lentils. Spinach, white beans, fortified cereals, and shellfish are also great choices.

Love your legumes: Eat to beat diabetes

Ready for some surprisingly good news? Eating lentils and other legumes may just keep type 2 diabetes at bay.

That's according to Spanish researchers who tracked the diets and health of several thousand adults. None of them had diabetes at the start of the four-year study, but they were at risk for cardiovascular problems.

The scientists discovered that the people who ate the most legumes had a lower risk of developing diabetes. And the winner among the different types of legumes? Lentils, of course. In fact, those who ate the most lentils were 33% less likely to get diabetes. And it didn't take a lot to get such results. They ate just one serving a week!

The researchers attribute the results in part to the high amounts of fiber in lentils and other legumes. All that roughage keeps you full longer, which helps keep your weight in check. That's important because obesity increases your risk of diabetes.

Just think — a 1/2 cup of cooked lentils provides nearly 8 grams of fiber. That's almost 40% of the amount senior women need each day, and more than a quarter of what older men should get.

In addition, lentils have a low glycemic index. Unlike, say, russet potatoes or white rice, lentils don't cause your blood sugar levels to rise quickly and then drop just as fast. Medical professionals believe that over time, these constant glucose surges and plummets can lead to insulin resistance and diabetes.

 Kitchen hacks

Cooking lentils is easy. No pre-soaking is required, and they usually take around 20 minutes or less to cook. Here's what to do.

- Determine how much you need. Dry lentils roughly double in volume when cooked.

- Check for any small stones by placing the lentils on a flat surface, such as a baking sheet. Rinse the legumes in a collander.

- Combine the lentils with water or broth in a pot. For 1 cup of dry lentils, you'll need 3 cups of liquid.

- Bring to a boil, cover tightly, and simmer until tender. Drain and serve.

Remember, never cook lentils in salted water as it will make them tough. And acidic ingredients, like tomatoes, will slow the cooking time.

Psst ... what's the skinny on lentils? They fight fatty liver

When it comes to protein-packed superfoods, you just can't beat the lentil. First off, it's loaded with lutein, an all-natural compound that's been found to boost the eyesight of folks with age-related macular degeneration. And they're nearly fat free, which can help you lose weight.

Here's something else most people don't know. Lentils are good for your liver.

Hard to believe, but not all liver problems are linked to drinking too much alcohol. Millions of Americans who drink little to no liquor have a condition called nonalcoholic fatty liver disease (NAFLD). In fact, it's estimated that around 25% of adults in the U.S. suffer from it.

Lentils come in many colors, from brown and yellow to red and green. But if you're looking for something extra special, you'll want to try black lentils. Dubbed the beluga, these tiny legumes look like caviar. They're nutty in flavor and have a firm skin, making them perfect in cold salads.

The main characteristic of this condition? Too much fat stored in the liver cells. If left untreated long enough, scarring and liver failure can occur. According to the American Liver Foundation, the following conditions increase the likelihood of developing NAFLD.

- being overweight or obese
- suffering from type 2 diabetes
- having high cholesterol

Enter the lentil. Scientists studied the diets of adults newly diagnosed with NAFLD and compared them with the foods eaten by people without the condition. The researchers found that the folks who ate lots of lentils and other legumes were less likely to develop the disease.

It makes sense when you consider that legumes are associated with slimmer waistlines, lower blood glucose levels, and improved cholesterol numbers.

But don't stop there. Separate research has found that the Mediterranean diet is the most effective eating plan for reducing the risk factors for NAFLD. You've probably already guessed that lentils are a big part of the diet, which also includes lots of fresh fruits and veggies, whole grains, nuts and seeds, fish, and olive oil. So dig in!

 Bright idea

Is there a way to stretch your food budget while cutting saturated fat and boosting nutrition? You betcha!

It's a slam dunk if you replace ground beef with lentils. Making the switch is super easy when you're in the mood for burgers, tacos, sloppy Joes, meatloaf, or chili. Just be sure to use brown or green lentils. They have a mild taste, along with a texture close to cooked ground beef. These lentils also tend to retain their shape after cooking.

You can substitute 1 cup of dry lentils for every pound of ground beef you would normally use. You'll want to stir in salt, lemon juice, or vinegar only after the lentils have simmered. They'll absorb the seasoning perfectly. Oh — don't forget that lentils are also excellent additions to soups, stews, and curries. You just might find yourself going meatless more than once a week.

A closer look
Slow cookers

Flip through a 1970s cookbook and you'll likely spot a crock pot recipe for "Hawaiian" meatballs in canned pineapple chunks and barbecue sauce. Then there's this one — pork chops slow cooked in condensed cream of mushroom soup. Talk about a heart attack on a plate.

Thank goodness the culinary world has evolved since then. While the crock pot has always been convenient — just drop in the ingredients, cover, and simmer away — it can also make tasty and nutritious meals for pennies on the dollar.

Focus on health. Did you know that slow cooking helps protect the nutrients in your food from being destroyed? That's super important if you're trying to eat right. And the crock pot is perfectly suited for cooking one of the healthiest sources of protein — dried beans.

Just toss them into your slow cooker and add stock and any other ingredients you want. Crock pot beans can fly solo, but they also add tons of flavor and texture to soup, chili, rice, and burritos.

Target your taste buds. You can make any slow-cooked recipe lip-smackin' good with a few simple tricks. For starters, saute veggies like onions, garlic, celery, and carrots before tossing them into the crock pot. Doing so maximizes the flavor. And if your recipe calls for meat, sear it first. The tasty crust boosts the savory goodness.

Meanwhile, you'll want to use dried herbs when slow cooking. Their pungency flourishes in the highly moist environment. Save fresh herbs for a garnish when serving.

Stretch that dollar. Your crock pot is a win-win for both your belly and your bottom line. First off, a long, slow cook makes cheaper cuts of meat — chuck roasts, pork shoulders, and chicken thighs — incredibly tender. Not so with the more expensive fare.

Slow cookers also use a lot less energy than electric ovens. And you won't be tempted to eat out as much knowing a hot, nutritious dinner is waiting for you on the kitchen counter. Think of all the savings on your utility and restaurant bills.

Peanuts

3 reasons to reach for this crowd-pleaser

You'll find them in a tin of mixed nuts, but as edible seeds that grow in pods, peanuts are actually part of the legume family. The surprises don't stop there. This popular snack is also full of nutrients that help maintain your weight, control blood sugar levels, and support heart health.

Go nuts to prevent unwanted pounds. Even though peanuts are calorie- and fat-dense, research shows that people who eat them don't tend to gain more weight than people who avoid them. Replace less healthy snacks with 1/2 ounce, or just about 2 tablespoons, of peanuts and you could prevent weight gain over the years.

This might be because they are so satisfyingly packed with fats, protein, and fiber that help you feel full for longer. Protein in peanuts is also a muscle builder. More muscle mass leads to a higher metabolism, making it easier to keep unwanted pounds at bay. Muscle mass declines as you age, so getting enough protein is vital for keeping you strong and fit.

Balance blood sugar with a smart swap. A simple switch by replacing higher carbohydrate foods with peanuts can help balance blood sugar levels. A recent study published in the journal *Nutrients* looked at people with diabetes who were put on a low-carbohydrate diet that replaced some starchy foods with peanuts. After three months, their blood sugar levels went down.

Instead of processed, carb-dense snacks like potato chips or candy bars, try a handful of peanuts or some peanut butter with fresh, high-fiber apple slices or hydrating, crunchy celery sticks. You'll satisfy cravings, and your blood sugar will stay more steady.

Healthy fats in peanuts boost heart health. Snacking on peanuts can do wonders for your heart. An analysis of studies showed that for every weekly serving — about an ounce — of nuts as part of a healthy diet, the risk of dying from heart disease dropped by about 8%. Likely because peanuts are packed with unsaturated fats, L-arginine, minerals, phenolic compounds, and phytosterols, all of which support heart health.

In fact, some of these nutrients, particularly the monounsaturated and polyunsaturated fats, help lower high blood pressure and high cholesterol, keeping your blood vessels clear and healthy.

 Boost the benefits

Peanut butter comes in various styles and textures. Whether you like smooth, chunky, or all-natural, there's a jar for you. However, not all peanut butter is created equal when it comes to nutrition.

First off, unless your spread contains at least 90% peanuts, it's not technically peanut butter, according to the Food and Drug Administration. More nuts mean more protein, fiber, and vitamin E. Enriched versions contain additional vitamins and minerals added during processing, boosting nutrition.

Some ingredients to check for and avoid are added sugar, corn syrup, and salt, often found in familiar brands. Keep added sugars under 3 grams per serving. All-natural "just peanuts" spread is ideal. You'll get all the nutrients with no additives. Don't pick a low-fat option since those will remove good fats.

While peanuts contain these heart-healthy fats, you'll want to avoid ingredients like palm oil that add unhealthy fats to your spread.

Unconventional peanut products you should try now

Major League Baseball fans eat 4 to 7 million bags of peanuts in a typical season, reports *Sports Illustrated*. Wowza. Sure, these game-day staples are legendary, but if you're only eating them salted and roasted, you're missing out. Learn how this incredible nut transforms into other culinary must-haves.

A flavorful, high-protein baking ingredient. Did you know there's a delicious, protein-packed flour that tastes like your favorite nut spread? Peanut flour is a healthy and tasty option made from roasted peanuts. It's perfect for special diets since it's gluten free and vegan.

The fats in peanuts are mostly removed to make flour, turning it into a concentrated source of protein with 10 to 15 grams per ounce and nutrients like folate, zinc, potassium, fiber, magnesium, phosphorus, and niacin. This process extends the shelf life and makes cooking with peanut flour a wise choice. Not only can you bake up yummy treats, but you can also use it as a thickener for sauces, stews, curries, smoothies, and more.

Pay attention to labels on powdered peanut butter. The first ingredient in many of these products is peanut flour, but manufacturers often go a step further and add other things like salt, sugar, and flavorings. The brands that contain 100% peanuts can make a healthy addition to smoothies or oatmeal, providing plenty of protein.

> Natural peanut butter separates easily. It's still perfectly safe to eat, but can be tricky to stir. Mix and store the container upside down. Next time you use it, flip it upright. Repeat this each use to prevent separation. Or mix and store it in the fridge where separation won't occur.

Bottom line — read the label. Some sellers use the terms powdered peanut butter and peanut flour interchangeably, but not always.

Peanut oil is what's missing from your pantry. It's healthier than many other types of oil. You can find it refined, roasted, and cold-pressed, each with different uses.

Refined peanut oil, for example, has a neutral flavor and high smoke point for frying. It's generally considered safe for people with peanut allergies since processing removes the allergens. Roasted oil, sometimes called gourmet, is more flavorful. It's used as a finishing oil because of the low smoke point.

No surprise that unrefined oils, like cold-pressed peanut oil, retain more nutrients than refined varieties. So weigh the pros and cons before buying.

 Kitchen hacks

A long-time lunchbox staple, peanut butter is creamy, rich, and delicious in both savory and sweet dishes.

- Punch up the flavor of soups, sauces, dressings, and curries with a dollop of your favorite spread. Serve on noodles, salads, and rice.
- Marinate chicken or pork with peanut butter, soy sauce, garlic, and ginger.
- Replace the tahini in hummus with peanut butter for a twist on this healthy bean dip.
- Pizza with chicken and bell peppers tastes other-worldly with a peanut butter drizzle.
- Oatmeal becomes a dreamy treat with a scoop of peanut butter and raspberries.
- Chili gains depth of flavor with a spoonful of this nut butter.
- Smoothies will stick to your ribs when you add healthy fats in the form of peanut butter
- Popcorn with a sprinkle of salt and peanut butter becomes a satisfying snack.

Soybeans

News you can use — take this superfood to heart

Folks have been eating soybeans for thousands of years, but Americans only started planting this crop in the 1800s. Fast forward a couple of centuries and you'll find that the U.S. produces just about half of the soybeans in the world.

Here's something else you might not know about these versatile legumes. They're one of the few vegetarian sources of protein that contain all the amino acids you need in your diet. Nifty, huh? But their health benefits don't stop there.

In fact, eating soy-based products may lower your risk of coronary heart disease. It's one of the reasons you'll want to dig into tofu — a food made from pressing curdled soy milk into blocks. A huge study of some 200,000 people found that those who ate at least one serving of tofu a week had an 18% lower risk of developing heart disease than those who ate less than that.

Tofu was, in part, particularly effective in postmenopausal women who weren't on hormone replacement therapy. A possible reason why? It's chock-full of isoflavones, plant compounds that mimic the effects of estrogen — a hormone that can help keep your blood vessels supple and blood pressure low.

Soooy good: Don't miss out on this tasty fare

Along with tofu, you'll want to try these other soy-based foods.

Edamame. Boil or steam the pods, and eat the nutty and buttery beans as is. You can also add them to stir-fries.

Miso. This seasoning paste is made from fermenting grains and soybeans. Miso goes great in marinades, sauces, and soups. Known for its salty and savory flavor, some miso can have a slightly spicy or sweet flavor.

Soy milk. This beverage is easy to make. Just blend soaked soybeans with water and then strain and boil the liquid. Soy milk typically has a mild flavor and is creamy in texture.

Soy nuts. You can mix up this popular snack by soaking soybeans in water and then roasting or baking them. Sprinkle on a little cajun spice for extra flavor.

Soy sauce. This salty condiment comes from fermenting soybeans and wheat. Its flavor and texture vary, depending upon production methods.

Tempeh. With a nutty, almost mushroom-like flavor, tempeh makes a good meat substitute. It's made by pressing fermented, cooked soybeans into a block.

Drink your way to better kidney health

Soy milk is a solid choice for folks who have suffered from kidney stones. That's because, compared with some other plant milks, it's not high in oxalates. Those are the compounds that combine with calcium to form the most common type of kidney stone.

Folks with a history of kidney stones shouldn't have more than 50 milligrams (mg) of oxalates a day.

A cup of soy milk provides less than 10 mg, compared with more than 27 mg in almond milk and 17 mg in cashew milk.

Other good low-oxalate choices are hemp, oat, macadamia, and rice milks.

When it comes to breast cancer, take a second look at soy

People used to think that eating soy increased the risk of breast cancer. It's easy to understand why, but luckily those days are in the past.

So where did the idea come from? Simple enough. Compounds in soy called isoflavones are plant estrogens. And, high levels of the female hormone estrogen have been linked to breast cancer.

> It's hard to beat soy milk for a healthy treat. A single cup has more fiber, iron, niacin, and vitamin B12 than a cup of low-fat cow's milk. Soy milk is also lower in sugar, and has roughly the same amount of calcium and vitamin D as its dairy cousin.

Here's why it's OK to eat soy. According to the Mayo Clinic, the compounds in soy-based foods don't contain high enough levels of estrogen to increase the risk of breast cancer. In fact, studies suggest that a lifelong, soy-rich diet reduces women's risk of developing this disease.

However, the same can't be said for soy supplements. They contain much higher isoflavone concentrations than good old soybeans.

Of course, you'll want to consult with your doctor before changing your diet. But it's safe to say that it's healthier to favor primary soy products — edamame, tempeh, miso, soy milk, and unsweetened soy yogurt, for example — over processed options.

Achieve a healthier brain through your stomach

When you eat soy, you're doing far more than enjoying a tasty treat. For starters, soy-based foods are an excellent source of unsaturated fats. That makes this mighty legume a fantastic replacement for meats, dairy, and oils high in unhealthy saturated fats.

But soybeans offer even more benefits. In fact, they may keep your brain healthy as you age.

Lowers dementia risk. Ever hear of white matter lesions? They're abnormal tissues on the brain that appear as bright white spots on brain scans. These lesions are associated with cognitive decline and dementia.

But help may be on the way. That's what researchers found after measuring the amount of equol in the blood of some 90 older adults with normal cognition. Equol is a substance with antioxidant properties that forms when your gut bacteria metabolize soy.

The seniors underwent brain scans between six and nine years later. And the results were astonishing.

"We found 50% more white matter lesions in people who cannot produce equol compared to people who can produce it, which is a surprisingly huge effect," says Dr. Akira Sekikawa, associate professor of epidemiology at the University of Pittsburgh Graduate School of Public Health.

Not everybody can make equol. A lot depends on the type of gut bacteria you have. But Dr. Sekikawa hopes to evaluate the protective effects of equol supplements. So stay tuned!

Keeps depression at bay. Here's an added bonus to eating more soybeans. They're just loaded with an amino acid called tryptophan. And recent research indicates that a tryptophan-rich diet protects against depression.

How's that? Tryptophan is needed to make serotonin, a chemical that carries messages between nerve cells in your brain. And you guessed it — low levels of serotonin have been linked to depression.

Gorgeous skin starts here

Have you noticed that your skin is drier, thinner, and less elastic? If that's the case, aging may be taking its toll. But there's one easy way to reduce these effects — eat soy-based foods.

That's what scientists found after giving a group of postmenopausal women a concentrated soy extract for six months.

Afterwards, they measured the women's skin and found that the treatment improved skin thickness, and also increased concentrations of collagen and elastic fibers.

It made sense to perform this study on women who had already gone through menopause. After all, they had already experienced big drops in their estrogen levels. Those hormonal changes can really affect your skin, making it prone to thinning, wrinkling, and sagging. In fact, several studies have shown that estrogen therapy helps increase skin thickness in senior women.

And here's how soy comes to the rescue. It's chock-full of isoflavones, a natural plant chemical that works in ways similar to estrogen. So load up on soybeans — they're by far the most concentrated source of isoflavones.

Here's some other exciting news. Soy — and its isoflavones — applied to the skin can also make it look younger. So try this recipe for hydrating success. Mix 4 tablespoons of soy milk with 2 teaspoons of nutmeg powder and 2 teaspoons of plain Greek yogurt.

Massage the mixture into your skin for a minute or so. Wait another moment and then rinse with lukewarm water. Pat dry and you're done!

 Watch out

Do you ever get headaches, chest pains, or other symptoms after eating foods prepared with monosodium glutamate (MSG)? Restaurants love to use this flavor enhancer, and it also shows up a lot in processed foods.

If you are sensitive to MSG, you may want to stay away from soy products. That's because they're naturally high in the amino acid glutamate. According to the Food and Drug Administration, the glutamate in MSG is chemically indistinguishable from the glutamate that's naturally present in food.

Other foods containing high amounts of this amino acid include Parmesan cheese, fish sauce, tomatoes, walnuts, and processed meats.

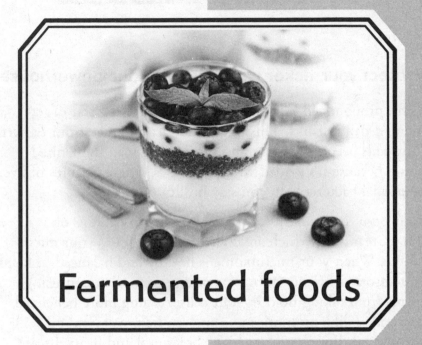

Fermented foods

Kefir

Protect your ticker with this probiotic powerhouse

Kefir, pronounced kuh-FEAR, may be the rising star of fermented dairy drinks. This tangy and tart beverage from Eastern Europe is becoming more and more popular in the United States because it's loaded with probiotics. These cultures of live, beneficial bacteria help you stay healthy.

Your body, particularly your gut, is home to trillions of microorganisms, which are collectively known as your microbiome. When your microbiome is healthy and balanced, it helps you absorb nutrients from food and prevent disease-causing germs from taking hold in your cells. Adding more beneficial bacteria — like probiotics — can even help you fend off chronic conditions such as high cholesterol and heart disease.

A fizzy, yogurt-like refreshment to curb your cholesterol. Nearly 2 out of every 5 Americans have high cholesterol. This dangerous condition can cause waxy, fatty buildups in arteries, which increase the risk of heart attacks and strokes. There's good news, though. Researchers think kefir can help keep cholesterol levels from getting out of control.

In a small study, overweight women who drank four servings of kefir a day had lower cholesterol levels than a control group after eight weeks. One theory as to why this fermented beverage is so powerful? Another paper suggests probiotics can help lower the amount of cholesterol your gut absorbs.

This creamy drink may reduce your heart attack risk. Experts estimate that nearly 805,000 Americans have a heart attack every year. And even scarier, they think 20% of those people don't even realize they had one. Adding plenty of probiotic-rich foods like kefir to your diet is a great way to protect your ticker.

Researchers recently published a study in the *British Journal of Nutrition* that examined the heart health and dairy habits of 2,000 men for five years. They found that men who ate a lot of fermented dairy products — like kefir and yogurt — had a lower risk of heart attacks.

The same wasn't true for those who ate a lot of unfermented dairy. Scientists think benefits may be due to certain compounds that are formed during the fermentation process.

 Kitchen hacks

Tired of simply drinking kefir? Try these creative ways to indulge in this dairy delight.

- Blend it into a smoothie with your favorite fruits and greens for a probiotic-rich snack.

- Fill popsicle molds with kefir and chopped fruit for a sweet summertime treat.

- Replace the milk in your cereal with kefir to add a nice tang to your morning meal.

- Enjoy it in a homemade salad dressing. Just mix kefir with your favorite ingredients. Parsley, lemon juice, garlic, olive oil, pepper — you name it.

Follow these simple steps to make your own kefir

Whipping up your own batch of kefir is so easy, you'll be wondering why you haven't been doing it for years. As an added bonus, the homemade stuff packs in even more probiotics than store-bought brands because it doesn't have to be processed to survive the trip to the supermarket. Here's what you'll need to get started.

- Starter cultures. Many people prefer to use clusters of yeast and bacteria called kefir grains, because you can strain them out and use them again to make another batch. You'll find dried kefir starter grains online or in some health food stores. Simply follow the manufacturer's instructions to activate them so they're ready for fermenting. Starter powders are also available at stores and online, but one packet will only make a single batch.

- Dairy milk. Avoid anything labeled "ultra-high temperature pasteurized" or else it won't ferment properly.

- A clean, glass jar or bottle, such as a mason jar.

Ready to get started? Combine 1 cup of milk with 1 teaspoon of active kefir grains in your glass jar. For powdered starters, use the measurements on the packet.

Cover the top with cheesecloth or a paper towel and secure it with a rubber band. Do not place an airtight lid on this. As the milk ferments, it will produce gasses that can cause pressure to build up in a closed bottle. If this pressure gets too high, the bottle may explode.

Let it sit for about 24 hours at room temperature, checking in every few hours. It will be finished when the milk has reached the consistency of heavy cream and the resulting beverage tastes tangy. The kefir may separate into thick and watery layers if it sits for too long.

If you're using grains, strain them out and put them into a cup of milk to start a new batch. If you don't want to make more kefir straight away, you can store them covered tightly in the fridge for up to a month. The finished kefir will keep in the fridge for up to one week if you keep it covered with a snug-fitting lid.

A closer look
Prebiotics

It's like a hidden jungle in there. Trillions of tiny organisms interacting with each other in your gut. But don't be scared. These guys help you absorb nutrients and keep your immune system strong. So why not give them a helping hand? That's where prebiotics come in. This term refers to various fibers and other naturally occurring compounds that feed the helpful bacteria living in your digestive tract.

Fiber versus prebiotics — what's the difference? Your body can't digest all of the nutrients in the food you eat. The carbohydrates that pass through your digestive system without breaking down are often called fibers. While your body may not be able to absorb fiber, the bacteria and other microorganisms living in your gut use certain ones — known as prebiotics — for fuel.

So how do you know if the fiber in a food is a prebiotic? The five main types are inulin, galactooligosaccharides (GOS), fructooligosaccharides (FOS), oligofructose (OF), and chicory fiber. If you're buying a prebiotic supplement or scanning the label of packaged foods, look out for these nutrients.

Foods high in prebiotics. Experts estimate that you need to get around 3 to 5 grams of prebiotic fibers every day in order to properly fuel your gut microbiome. Pile your plate high with the following foods to make sure you're getting enough nutrients.

- apples
- bananas
- chicory root
- flaxseed
- Jerusalem artichokes
- garlic
- oats
- onions

You can also check your local grocery store for breads, yogurts, or cereals that have been fortified with prebiotics.

When to avoid these special fibers. Digestive woes? You may want to be careful about adding prebiotics to your daily diet. Because prebiotics are fiber, suddenly adding too many to your meals could cause digestive discomfort, bloating, and gas. If you have irritable bowel syndrome or want to follow a low-FODMAP (fermentable oligosaccharides, disaccharides, monosaccharides, and polyols) diet, then prebiotics may not be for you.

Kimchi

2 ways this fantastic fermented food will help you dodge diabetes

Kimchi is a staple in nearly every Korean meal. In fact, this fiery, naturally fermented dish is so popular that when South Korea sent its first astronaut to space, a specially designed container packed with kimchi tagged along.

In the past few years, the rest of the world has started to catch on to why this spicy cabbage dish is so popular in Korea. In addition to its unique flavor, kimchi is packed with probiotics and other nutrients that could help you stay fit and healthy for years to come. Some studies even suggest that this powerful fermented food might hold the key to helping prevent blood sugar spikes and diabetes.

Beat the blood sugar blues by the cupful. In a small study, researchers recruited 100 healthy young adults and asked them to follow a strict diet for one week. The volunteers were then either assigned to a high-kimchi diet or a low-kimchi diet. At the end of the study, researchers found that the people who stuck to a high-kimchi diet had much better fasting glucose levels than the other group. As an added bonus, those who ate more kimchi also had better cholesterol levels.

That's great news for people who are at risk of diabetes. If you have high levels of fasting glucose, your odds of developing type 2 diabetes go up. Want to try it yourself? People in the high-kimchi group ate a little less than 1 1/2 cups of kimchi a day.

Melt away the fat with this tangy treat. Carrying around too much extra weight dramatically increases your chances of diabetes.

Experts estimate that people with obesity are six times more likely to get diabetes than those who are at a healthy weight. Here's why.

Your body normally stores glucose — which it uses for energy — in the liver. However, if you have too many fat cells packed into your liver, there's nowhere for all the extra glucose to go. Instead, it stays in the bloodstream and causes your pancreas to become overworked and eventually less effective at making the insulin you need to process glucose.

Fortunately, kimchi may help you shed those extra pounds. In a small study, South Korean researchers found that overweight people who ate fermented kimchi showed reductions in body fat and fasting blood sugar.

 Watch out

On a low-salt diet? You need to be careful about chowing down on kimchi and many other fermented veggies. The fermentation process uses high levels of salt in order to preserve the cabbage and promote the growth of helpful, friendly bacteria. That means some kimchi can be nearly 3% salt by weight. So a single half-cup serving could clock in with more than half of your daily recommended sodium intake.

If you're after probiotics but have high blood pressure or other reasons to limit salt in your diet, consider taking probiotic supplements or eating low-salt fermented foods instead. Otherwise, read the nutrition label of any kimchi you buy and be mindful of your sodium intake.

Pile your plate high with kimchi to load up on this vital vitamin

About 2 out of every 3 men over the age of 70 don't get enough vitamin K in their diets, according to one study. That's bad news because this nutrient plays an important role in preventing heart disease and brittle bones.

Don't worry, though. You can make sure you don't run low on vitamin K by eating plenty of kimchi. A mere half cup of this nutritional powerhouse has 33 micrograms (mcg) of vitamin K. That goes a long way toward getting the 120 mcg recommended for men and 90 mcg for women, as well as scoring these benefits.

Safeguard your blood vessels. In a recent, 23-year study of over 53,000 people, scientists found that those who ate the most foods rich in vitamin K1 — the kind found in vegetables — had a 21% lower chance of hospitalization due to stroke or other cardiovascular problems than the people who didn't get much vitamin K in their diets.

"We believe that vitamin K works by protecting against the calcium buildup in the major arteries of the body," says senior study author Nicola Bondonno, Ph.D.

Support your bones. Your body grows a whole new skeleton every 10 years or so. Bit by bit, the cells in your bones break down and your body needs to build them back up. If you don't have the proper nutrients, however, you can't rebuild a strong, healthy frame. This can lead to a disease called osteoporosis, which is marked by brittle bones and an increased risk of fractures. One of the most important nutrients to keep your body stocked with? Vitamin K. Running low on this nutrient is linked to a higher risk of fractures.

Can't stand the heat? Top tips to cool the burn

Kimchi is traditionally loaded with chili peppers. That's what gives it a blazing, red color. While the fermentation process tones down the heat, this dish can still pack quite a punch. So if you bought a batch of kimchi that's just a bit too spicy for your taste, don't throw it out. These pointers can help you cool the heat and salvage your kimchi.

- Add a pinch of something sweet. Sugar or honey can help tone down spicy foods. Mix it in slowly and taste it frequently, or else you may wind up making your dinner taste like a dessert.

- Serve it alongside something starchy, like rice, pasta, or bread. These can help bulk out the meal and cut down on fiery flavors.

- Tame the heat with a dollop of dairy. Yogurt, milk, and other dairy products bind to the chemical in hot peppers that makes your tongue burn.

- A splash of acid can neutralize the heat. Adding a tiny bit of lemon juice or vinegar helps brighten up flavors and cool down spicy foods.

 Kitchen hacks

Calling all kimchi newbies. Use these tips to make the most of this delicious delicacy.

- Decide what type of kimchi you want. While it's usually made with cabbage, "kimchi" can mean any kind of naturally fermented Korean pickle. Some well-stocked stores may have options made from other veggies like daikon radish, mustard leaf, or green onions.

- Read the label. Look for unpasteurized kimchi if you want to get the most beneficial bacteria.

- Buy refrigerated kimchi and store it in the fridge. The cold temp slows down fermentation so it doesn't go bad as fast. It will keep for up to six months, as long as there is no mold in the jar.

Kombucha

Antioxidant power: Check out the budding benefits of this tangy tea

Kombucha, pronounced kom-BOO-cha, has been around for thousands of years. This fermented, slightly fizzy beverage likely originated in ancient China before slowly spreading across the world. Its reported health benefits have made it a mainstay in nearly every grocery store in America. In fact, experts estimate sales of this exotic drink topped $1 billion recently, and the market is still growing.

So what makes this ancient drink so popular? It's made from high-antioxidant black, green, white, and oolong teas. And new research shows that the fermentation process increases its antioxidant powers.

Bolster your mind and boost your mood with this delightful drink. Feeling blue? Reach for a glass of kombucha. Studies suggest that the naturally occurring antioxidants in tea called polyphenols might help fend off inflammation in the brain that's associated with depression.

Experts also think these compounds could help protect your noggin against more than just mood disorders. Getting more polyphenols is linked to lower odds of developing dementia, including Alzheimer's disease. Because kombucha is loaded with these same compounds, it may have these benefits, too.

Sip on kombucha to curb your risk of cancer. Researchers think tea could offer up some powerful protection against cancer. Studies show that people who drink the most tea are often the least likely to develop certain cancers, such as breast and colon cancer. The polyphenols from this drink may stop cancer cells from replicating and spreading throughout the body.

Early evidence shows that kombucha may have similar perks. Test tube studies have found that kombucha is great at battling cancerous cells. However, human studies still need to be done, so keep your eyes out for more information in the future.

If your kombucha ferments or sits in the fridge too long, it can develop a strong vinegary tang. But you don't need to let it go to waste. Simply replace the vinegar in your favorite home-made salad dressing recipe with an equal amount of this fermented drink.

Spoiler alert! 3 surefire signs that it's time to toss the batch

Before kombucha was on the shelves of every major grocery store, enthusiasts and small vendors fermented batches of this refreshing beverage in their home kitchens. The process is fairly simple. All you need is tea, sugar, a starter, and time in order to make this sparkling, tangy, and slightly sweet drink.

While you can still find plenty of people who make their own kombucha, you may want to take caution before downing a glass of the homemade stuff. Experts warn that some kombucha could be harmful to your health. If something goes wrong during the fermentation process, it could become home to some dangerous bacteria, yeast, or fungi.

Another reason to be wary about DIY kombucha? It may be lightly alcoholic. Commercial products have less than 0.5% alcohol, but scientists say some home-brewed batches can contain up to 3% alcohol by volume. If you're sensitive to alcohol or have a compromised immune system, you should steer clear of kombucha.

That doesn't mean all kombucha is dangerous. If you're getting this drink from a friend or vendor, check for these signs of spoilage.

- Mold. You may see some sediment or other gel-like clumps floating in kombucha, but that isn't a cause for concern. However, any signs of fuzzy mold means you should avoid drinking that kombucha.

- Odd odor. Trust your nose. If the drink smells spoiled or too acidic, don't drink it.

- Overly vinegary taste. While good kombucha is slightly sour, if it tastes strongly of vinegar the drink is no longer good for sipping.

The Centers for Disease Control and Prevention says that 4 ounces of kombucha a day is safe for most people. Others say not to drink more than 12 ounces — or 1 1/2 cups — of kombucha a day. If you drink too much, it may lead to digestive issues or cause too much acid to build up in your bloodstream.

Simplify shopping with this easy advice

The kombucha craze is in full swing, and that means you get to choose among dozens of different flavors and brands. While it's nice to have options when you're shopping, it can be overwhelming if you're not sure what to look for. Fortunately, these top tips can make it easy to buy a refreshing drink.

- Stick to the refrigerated section. If you want your kombucha to be loaded with healthy, friendly microbes — known as probiotics — you'll need to look for one that is labeled raw or unpasteurized. This drink needs to be kept cold, so look for it with juice and other refrigerated beverages.

- Scan the label to avoid getting too much sugar. While kombucha will have some sugar from the fermentation process, some brands may add extra sweeteners or flavorings that can impact the health benefits.

Miso

2 ways this savory soup keeps your heart healthy

Need a warm, comforting bowl of soup? Forget the chicken noodle. Instead, try a helping of miso soup. This traditional, Japanese staple is satisfyingly savory, salty, and — even better — packed with nutrients that may be great for your ticker. Miso, a condiment made from fermented soybeans, might be just what you need to lower your blood pressure and resting heart rate.

Beat high blood pressure with help from an unlikely dish. Normally, salty foods are the last thing you'd think of if you're trying to combat hypertension. That's because your body hangs on to extra water to flush excess sodium out, which makes your heart and blood vessels work even harder. But miso may help counteract blood pressure spikes, even with the added sodium.

In a small study conducted by Japanese researchers, scientists recruited 40 people with high blood pressure and asked them to either eat miso soup or a regular, unfermented soy soup every day. At the end of eight weeks, the researchers discovered that miso — but not regular soy — led to lower nighttime blood pressure. And it didn't increase daytime blood pressure. The jury's out on why.

People in the study ate 32 grams of miso every day, which is about 2 tablespoons. If you have high blood pressure, talk to your doctor before adding more salt to your diet.

A soothing bowl of miso soup to calm your heart. Your ticker has to pump thousands of gallons of blood throughout your body every single day. The stronger your heart is, the easier it can move all that blood through your veins.

One of the simplest ways to know if your heart is functioning efficiently? Pay attention to your resting heart rate. A healthy adult heart will beat between 60 and 100 times every minute. In some cases, like elite athletes, that number may be in the low 40s.

If you wish to keep your heart rate lower, you may want to reach for the miso. Researchers published a study that linked eating miso soup frequently with having a lower resting heart rate. More studies are needed to know just how much miso you'd need to eat to get these benefits, so keep an eye out for future research.

 Watch out

Trying to stay gluten free? You may be surprised to find that not all miso pastes fit your diet. This condiment can be made from a variety of beans and grains. While soybeans and rice are by far the most common, it's not unusual for miso recipes to call for barley, wheat, or other grains.

Read the labels and ingredients list carefully when you're shopping for miso. Unless the product specifically says it is gluten free, don't assume that it doesn't contain any of these grains. And if you decide to opt for a pre-made miso soup mix, check that it doesn't contain soy sauce. This salty staple is often made with soybeans and wheat, so it isn't gluten free.

The best condiment to beef up your muscles

As you age, your body transforms. Your hair starts to change color, wrinkles appear in your skin, and your muscles lose some of their old strength. It may be subtle at first, but as your muscle mass wanes, you can develop sarcopenia. This condition puts you at risk of falls and fractures, and can take away your mobility.

If you have diabetes, you're more likely to develop this dreaded disease. Scientists aren't exactly sure why that's the case, but one theory is that high levels of glucose in your blood can cause your muscles to waste away.

There's good news, though. Regularly adding miso to your diet could help prevent sarcopenia from taking hold. In a recent paper in the journal *Nutrients*, researchers studied the diets of men and women with type 2 diabetes. They discovered that the women who regularly ate miso soup were less likely to develop sarcopenia.

The reason this condiment is so powerful? The study's authors think soy compounds that mimic estrogen help protect the body from accumulating too much fat and breaking down muscle.

Master miso with this simple shopping guide

Time to stock your fridge with miso. But each type has a distinct flavor and use, so you may not know what to buy. Here's how to pick which one is best for you.

- White (shiro) miso. Also known as mellow or sweet miso, this bean paste has the shortest fermentation time and lightest flavor. It's usually the least salty, too. Because of its mild taste, white miso is a great addition to salad dressings and marinades. You can also use it to add a savory punch in recipes that call for butter.

- Yellow (shinshu) miso. It has a slightly longer fermentation period than white miso, which gives it a more pronounced savory and nutty flavor. It's good for miso soup or to add a bit of extra flavor to long braises or marinades.

- Red (aka) miso. This miso can take well over a year to ferment. Because it spends so long developing its flavors, they're strong and very pronounced. It's a great option to complement other hearty flavors. Use it sparingly because it can easily outshine other ingredients.

- Barley (mugi) miso. While most miso is made from a mix of soybeans and other beans, you'll find some made with barley. Despite its darker color, this type has a lighter, sweeter taste similar to white miso.

You can generally store covered miso in the refrigerator for up to a year.

2 more must-try dishes to satisfy your soy cravings

Admit it. You're hooked on miso's savory flavor. Here's another couple of fermented soy foods that will have your taste buds asking for more.

- Tempeh. If you're on a low-sodium diet, or simply want a more filling food, this Indonesian bean cake may be just what you need. It's made by fermenting whole soybeans with a starter culture so it forms a little protein-rich cake that has a mild, slightly nutty flavor. It's great raw, but it can be steamed, sauteed, or stir-fried in any recipe instead of meat.

- Natto. This Japanese standby is often served with soy sauce and karashi mustard on a bed of rice. It's loaded with nutrients like vitamin K, calcium, and protein. However, this food has a sticky texture and strong flavor that some liken to an aged cheese, so it may be a bit of an acquired taste.

Sauerkraut

Friendliest foods to soothe your stomach

Experts estimate that microbes living in your body outnumber your own cells 10 to 1. More than 100 trillion bacteria, yeasts, and fungi — collectively known as your microbiome — live alongside you. They help your body digest food, fend off diseases, and produce vitamins and minerals important to your health. If the microbes in your gut aren't healthy, you can develop problems in your pipes.

One of the best ways to make sure you're keeping your microbiome in good shape? Add some helpful, healthy bacteria to your gut. Traditionally fermented foods, like sauerkraut, are loaded with friendly microbes known as probiotics.

This flavorful fare tackles IBS symptoms. Suffer from chronic bloating, gas, constipation, or diarrhea? You may have irritable bowel syndrome (IBS). Recently, scientists have found some evidence that this digestive disorder can be triggered by disturbances in the gut microbiome. Many sufferers develop an especially bad bout of tummy troubles after taking antibiotics or developing an infection that alters the bacteria in their guts.

Fortunately, fermented foods may help get the right bacteria back into your microbiome. In a small study, Norwegian researchers asked people with IBS to eat sauerkraut every day. The experts found that the addition helped alter the participants' gut bacteria, which led to fewer IBS symptoms.

Arm yourself with fermented foods to fight UC flare-ups. Ulcerative colitis (UC), an inflammatory bowel disease, can cause symptoms such as diarrhea, cramping, and rectal bleeding.

Letting it go unchecked for years could lead to severe complications. Think malnutrition, holes in your colon, and an increased risk of colorectal cancer. Uh-oh.

The good news? An analysis of 18 studies suggests that probiotics might bring relief from UC. However, more research needs to be done to determine exactly what strains of bacteria are most beneficial.

Subtle signs your favorite fermented food brand is second-rate

Sauerkraut has long been a staple in America. In fact, the first English mentions of this food on American soil date back to 1776. It should come as no surprise that you can find dozens of brands and varieties of this tangy treat at grocery stores. However, not all are created equal. Here are a few ways to avoid buying the wrong thing.

- Don't touch anything with vinegar on the label. If you want to get the most probiotic benefits out of your sauerkraut, you want to make sure it's truly fermented. The tangy flavor of real sauerkraut comes from the lactic acid created during the fermentation process and not other additives.

- Steer clear of fermented foods that have been canned or pasteurized. Heating the probiotics will kill them off and take away some of sauerkraut's health benefits. Only buy products stored in the refrigerated section.

How this sour treat can help you trim your waistline

A whopping 3 out of every 4 adults in America are overweight. Carrying around that spare tire is bad news in the long run.

Experts say that if you aren't at a healthy weight, you're at greater risk for heart disease, type 2 diabetes, high blood pressure, stroke, and many types of cancer.

If you want to drop a few pounds and melt away fat, don't turn to fad diets. Instead, make sure your meals are made up of the right foods. That doesn't mean you're stuck with boring fare. Jazz up your healthy dishes with sauerkraut. This nutritional power-house is loaded with probiotics that may help you slim down.

In a small study published in the journal *Obesity*, researchers asked young men to eat a high-fat, high-calorie diet along with either a placebo or a probiotic supplement that contained various strains including *Lactobacillus plantarum*, which is common in sauerkraut. The study revealed that the people who took probiotics gained less body mass and fat than those who took the placebo.

Need another reason to add sauerkraut to your meals? This dish is a great source of fiber without being high in calories. A cup contains 4 grams of fiber, which will help keep you feeling full so you don't overeat.

Want to boost your mood and sharpen your mind? Start with your gut

Ancient Greek physicians believed that disruptions in your gut could lead to mental illness. Now, modern scientists think there may be some truth to this wisdom.

Your intestinal tract can send signals to your brain, and vice versa. That means inflammation and imbalances in your gut microbiome may contribute to stress, anxiety, depression, and even dementia. Fortunately, fermented food could hold the key to keeping your gut, and in turn your mind, in top shape.

Add sauerkraut to your plate to lift your spirits. Looking for comfort food? Your first instinct may be to reach for sugary sweets or salty, savory snacks, but there's something better you can eat to soothe your mood. A helping of sauerkraut might be the secret to fending off depression.

Korean researchers studied the diets of over 26,000 people and found that probiotic-rich foods are associated with a lower risk of depression in men. The exact cause is unclear, but one of the theories is that probiotics can help suppress inflammation in the gut that is often linked with mood disorders such as depression.

Slash dementia odds with the right foods. Changes in your gut microbiome could be linked to an increased risk of dementia, according to new research from Japanese scientists. They examined the microbiomes of people with dementia and compared them to similar, but healthy, volunteers. People with high levels of lactic acid — which is produced with the help of friendly bacteria like *Lactobacillus* and *Bifidobacteria* — were less likely to have dementia.

And early research suggests that taking probiotics or eating fermented foods could help protect people from cognitive decline. Exactly how much you should eat or which strains of probiotics you'd need to take is still unclear. In the meantime, it's best to add plenty of naturally fermented foods, like sauerkraut, to your meals.

2 ways this dish amps up immunity by the forkful

Feel a cold coming on? It may be time to pile your plate high with sauerkraut. This traditionally fermented dish is a great way to boost your body's natural defenses against germs. The secret lies in two of the most important nutrients hidden away in this underrated delicacy.

Load up on vitamin C with a surprising source. Famed explorer Captain Cook managed to keep scurvy from plaguing his crews by making sure they all loaded up on sauerkraut. Though Cook didn't know it at the time, this fermented cabbage dish is packed with vitamin C. A single cup offers 14% to 17% of your daily needs.

Research shows that getting plenty of this vitamin can help your immune system repel disease-causing germs, too. Men should get at least 90 milligrams (mg) of vitamin C every day, and women need 75 mg.

Call on friendly bacteria to crowd out any invaders. Keeping your gut microbiome healthy and balanced is an important way to prevent disease from running rampant in your body. While it may seem odd to eat foods loaded with live cultures of active bacteria to stop yourself from getting sick, don't worry.

Probiotics are bacteria that aren't harmful to your body, unlike disease-causing germs. If you have a community of strong, friendly bacteria in your gut, they can help prevent their dangerous cousins from breaching your body's immune system.

 Watch out

You need to look out for certain foods if you're prone to migraines. And unfortunately, fermented foods can be one of the worst offenders. That's because sauerkraut, kimchi, and other probiotic-rich foods often pack a double whammy of common migraine triggers.

- Tyramine. This compound occurs naturally in many protein-rich foods as well as fermented things, such as sauerkraut or aged cheeses.

- Salt. Traditionally, the fermentation process uses salt to ensure dangerous bacteria don't spoil the food as it ferments. However, foods high in sodium are known to encourage headaches.

Migraine triggers vary from person to person. If you notice that you get headaches after eating sauerkraut, consider talking to your doctor about taking probiotic supplements instead.

A closer look
Fermentation and probiotics

Still have some things you want to know about loading up on fermented foods and healthy bacteria? The answers to these common questions can help you unravel a few more mysteries about the tangy treats.

Do my pickles contain probiotics? Grocery store pickles share many similarities with the naturally fermented foods — such as sauerkraut and kimchi — that are chock-full of beneficial bacteria. Both are veggies that have been preserved in a salty brine. However, most of the pickled foods you'll find in the grocery store have been preserved in a solution of vinegar, sugar, and salt, and don't have any probiotics in them. You may be able to find fermented pickles in the refrigerated section, though. Look for ones that have only salt, water, vegetables, and whole spices on the ingredient label.

Can I ferment foods at home? Making homemade kimchi, sauerkraut, or other fermented foods is a common practice. But if it's not something you're familiar with, you need to be careful. Improperly fermented foods carry the risk of causing dangerous foodborne illnesses such as botulism.

If you want to try fermenting, find a reliable recipe and follow all the steps closely so you don't grow dangerous bacteria. The National Center for Home Food Preservation has recipes and guides online at *nchfp.uga.edu/how/can6a_ferment.html* that can help you get started correctly.

What should I look for in a probiotic supplement? You may opt for a probiotic pill instead of eating fermented foods if you're watching your sodium intake or have allergies. Choose a supplement with at least 1 billion colony forming units of live, active bacteria. Look for brands that contain well-studied strains of bacteria, such as *Lactobacillus* or *Bifidobacteria*.

Can I cook with fermented foods and still get all the health benefits? You may be tempted to add sauerkraut to your stew or mix a helping of chopped kimchi into a stir-fry, but heating the probiotic bacteria will destroy them and their health benefits. Instead, serve fermented foods on the side.

Yogurt

Steer clear of dangerous conditions with this fantastic food

Yogurt has been a staple dish in Central Asia for thousands of years. But it didn't make its way west until 1542, when the king of France came down with a nasty stomach bug that his doctors couldn't cure. That is, until the sultan of the Ottoman Empire sent the perfect antidote — yogurt.

It's a good thing, too. This superfood is packed with powerful nutrients that can keep you healthy.

Fight weak bones, forgetfulness, and high blood pressure with yogurt. A single cup of plain, low-fat yogurt provides nearly half the amount of bone-bolstering calcium that seniors need each day. This mighty mineral is a building block for your skeleton, which means you need plenty of it to prevent osteoporosis. Even better? Studies show that calcium can do a whole lot more.

- Improve your mind with a heaping helping of yogurt. A small Canadian study found that older women scored better on tests measuring attention, memory, and language after having eaten vitamin D- and calcium-fortified yogurt every day for three months.

- Running low on calcium could put your blood pressure in jeopardy. Your body uses this mineral to help your blood vessels tighten and relax on cue. Without enough calcium, it's harder for your heart to push blood through your veins and arteries. This increases your risk of developing dangerously high blood pressure.

Women over age 50 should get 1,200 milligrams of calcium a day. Men should get 1,000 milligrams until they turn 71, when they should increase that amount to 1,200 milligrams.

Probiotics tackle a number of health issues. Your body is home to nearly 5 pounds of microscopic organisms that help you digest food, battle disease, and even regulate your mood. Collectively, these tiny creatures are known as your microbiome. Each person has a unique mix of this bacteria.

Keeping a healthy balance of these microorganisms is an important part of staying fit and healthy. That's where probiotics come in. These microorganisms maintain or improve the health of the "good" bacteria in your body and make sure that the "bad" bacteria don't get the upper hand.

Yogurt is chock-full of these live cultures that, studies show, can help reduce weight, prevent type 2 diabetes, fortify the immune system, and soothe digestive issues. Probiotics can even fight bad breath by wiping out odor-causing bacteria in the mouth. So eat more yogurt to live your best life.

 Kitchen hacks

It's great to eat yogurt as a simple snack, in a smoothie, or as part of a healthy breakfast. But this tasty fare is even more versatile. Try these new ways to include yogurt in your diet.

- Mix your favorite herbs and spices with yogurt to make a simple, delicious marinade. The gentle acids in yogurt tenderize meat without turning it too tough or rubbery. As an added bonus, the yogurt turns into a crispy, flavorful crust when it's grilled or broiled.

- Whip up a low-fat salad dressing by adding fresh herbs, a dash of lemon or lime juice, and garlic to yogurt. This doubles as a dip for veggies, too.

- Swap mayonnaise with yogurt. Instead of using fatty mayo in potato salad or on a sandwich, opt for yogurt. This healthy alternative provides both creaminess and a zesty flavor — not to mention lots of protein.

Too many decisions? Get the scoop with this handy guide

Grocery store shelves are lined with dozens of flavors and brands of yogurts. How do you decide among them? You can't spend all day reading labels and tasting lots of samples to find the perfect product. But with a little know-how, you can select the perfect yogurt without worrying about buying the wrong kind.

> If you've ever seen antique brass pulls on bedroom dresser drawers, you know how this hardware can turn an unsightly black or green. Bring these handles back to their former glory by rubbing plain yogurt on them. Let them sit for a few hours before rinsing with water and buffing dry with a clean cloth.

- **Traditional yogurt.** This treat is made by heating milk to kill off any bad bacteria, and then adding cultures of *Lactobacillus* and *Streptococcus* bacteria that feast on the sugar in the milk and convert it into lactic acid. The result is a mild-flavored yogurt with a smooth, creamy texture. This type of yogurt works beautifully as a tasty substitute for milk or oil when baking.

- **Greek yogurt.** Confusingly, Greek yogurt isn't actually from Greece. Instead, companies marketed their strained yogurt as "Greek," and the name became synonymous with the process of filtering out whey. Because all that liquid is removed, this dairy product is tangier and thicker than traditional yogurt. Use in place of sour cream and any other high-fat creams when making sauces and dips.

- **Icelandic yogurt.** Also sold as Skyr, this product is made from skim milk and has a mild flavor. Even though it's sold with yogurt at most grocery stores, it's technically a cheese. That's because producers add rennet to the mix, allowing curds to form before the whey gets filtered out. The yogurt is repeatedly strained, resulting in a thicker, creamier texture than the Greek version. Icelanders enjoy Skyr with a sprinkling of berries and a tad of brown sugar.

- **Nondairy yogurt.** Skipping dairy doesn't mean you need to miss out on yogurt. Some supermarkets sell yogurt made from almond, soy, and other plant-based milks. Many are fortified with calcium and vitamin D so you won't be passing up these important nutrients. And most have the same probiotics you'll find in dairy-based yogurts. Look for brands with live active cultures.

 Watch out

The average American eats way too much added sugar — around 60 pounds of it a year. That's the weight of a healthy nine-year-old child. Yikes! All that sugar can increase your risk of heart disease, diabetes, and obesity.

Avoiding this ingredient may be a bit trickier than it seems. Manufacturers put sugar in lots of processed foods to boost flavor and extend shelf life. And it's lurking in places you might never expect — like in ketchup, barbecue sauce, and even yogurt. In fact, some sweetened yogurts contain more sugar than junk food.

If you're shopping for this dairy product, scan the label for the sugar content. The American Heart Association recommends that men limit their added sugar to 36 grams a day, while women shouldn't have more than 25 grams. Your best bet? Buy plain, unflavored yogurt and stir in fruit or a dash of vanilla extract.

A taste of hope: Eat this to dodge cancer

The human body is in a constant state of regeneration. In fact, you create an astounding 330 billion cells each day to replace others that have recently died off. But sometimes this process goes awry, which can lead to the uncontrolled growth of damaged cells into tumors.

Experts aren't exactly sure what triggers cancerous growths, or how to stop them. But research suggests that yogurt could help lower the risk of developing these two common cancers.

Probiotics help keep colon cancer at bay. A diet loaded with fat and processed meats could put you at prime risk for colon cancer. Slash the odds by eating yogurt instead.

Experts tracked colon cancer rates among 32,600 men and 55,700 women for nearly three decades. They also pulled information on their diets, lifestyles, and risk factors for the disease. The researchers found that the men who regularly ate at least two servings of yogurt a week had a 26% lower risk of developing precancerous growths.

The scientists think the probiotics in yogurt may be responsible. One theory they have is that these friendly microorganisms can help reduce inflammation in the colon, which is a major risk factor for cancer. Unfortunately, no association between yogurt and polyp risk was found in the women.

Lower the risk of breast cancer with yogurt. Breast cancer is one of the most common cancers in women. In fact, the Centers for Disease Control and Prevention estimates that 255,000 women in the United States are diagnosed with it each year. Taking every step you can to prevent this disease is vital.

A study published in *Current Developments in Nutrition* found that a high overall consumption of dairy products was linked to a significantly lower risk of breast cancer. Yogurt, in particular, stood out among the results, and was associated with a whopping 39% decrease in the women's chances of getting the disease.

Conversely, eating high amounts of cheddar and cream cheese was linked to a 53% increase in the chances of getting breast cancer. The researchers say further studies are needed to interpret the results of their study.

Out with gout — just pile on the dairy

Yogurt is a food that works wonders at fighting diabetes, high blood pressure, and infections. Turns out, it may also prevent gout.

This painful condition, caused by a buildup of uric acid that crystallizes, often affects the big toe. But it can show up in other joints, too. Fortunately, research suggests that eating low-fat yogurt and other dairy could keep gout from setting in.

Scientists tracked the diets of 47,150 men over 12 years. At the end of the study, they found that the participants who ate more dairy were less likely to get gout. The authors think the proteins in milk-based foods help reduce uric acid levels.

And unlike meat and seafood, dairy is low in compounds — called purines — that cause your body to produce uric acid. That means yogurt is a great way to get protein without increasing your risk of gout.

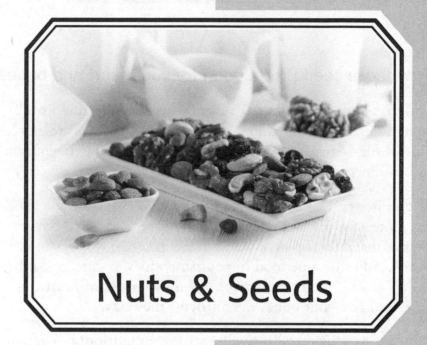

Nuts & Seeds

Chia seeds

Why these seeds are a boon for your heart and bones

You may remember chia seeds from Chia Pets, the cute little ceramic figurines containing chia sprouts that grow to resemble animal fur. Many Americans can instantly recall the jingle from old commercials — "Ch-ch-ch-chia!"

Today, however, researchers are finding that chia seeds are good for more than just fun decorations. They're nutritional power-houses that deliver potent health benefits for your heart and bones. Add this superfood to your smoothies, yogurt, and other dishes to lower your cholesterol, reduce your risk of heart disease, and give your bones the nutrients they crave.

Tiny seeds stuffed with two heart-loving nutrients. A recent review of 10 trials showed that eating chia seeds lowered "bad" LDL cholesterol and a type of fat found in the blood called triglycerides. At the same time, it increased "good" HDL cholesterol. How do these seeds support your ticker so well?

For starters, they're high in fiber, which works in your gut to drop the amount of cholesterol and fat that gets absorbed into your bloodstream. Chia seeds are also an excellent source of alpha-linolenic acid (ALA), an omega-3 fatty acid that helps cut your risk of cardiovascular disease.

Get your fill of bone-boosting minerals. If you want to load your plate with foods that can help you maintain a strong skeleton, you've hit the jackpot with chia seeds.

An ounce of these seeds — about 2 heaping tablespoons — contains 179 milligrams of calcium, or 15% to 18% of the amount you need each day. But even though calcium is famous for strengthening and repairing bones, it isn't the only mineral in chia seeds that fortifies your frame.

Tiny wonders they certainly are, but chia seeds can be dangerous if you don't soak them for at least five minutes before eating. To avoid choking, plump them up with enough liquid to allow them to expand. Skipping this step can allow the seeds to gel up in the esophagus, leading to an obstruction.

Manganese, phosphorus, and magnesium are involved in the structural development of your bones, too. An ounce of chia seeds boasts more than 20% of the recommended daily amount of each of these three minerals. Ch-ch-ch-cheers to that!

Can trendy chia banish belly fat?

Lose weight fast with chia water, claims a YouTube video with more than 7 million views. Is it just a fad, a trendy trick, or can drinking chia seeds soaked in a glass of water really help trim away unwanted fat? Research "weighs" in on just how effective these seeds are.

- A small study took a look at chia seeds and found that they have the potential to help you feel more full. Researchers asked participants to eat either chia seeds or flaxseeds. Those who ate chia reported a lower appetite.

- For overweight folks with type 2 diabetes, another study found that eating chia seeds may promote weight loss, maintain blood sugar control, and improve obesity-related risk factors. One group ate about 2 tablespoons of ground chia seeds each day, while the other had oat bran. Both followed a calorie-restricted diet. After six months, the chia seed group lost more weight and had a greater reduction in waist circumference, which is a measure of belly fat.

How is it that these oh-so-small seeds can help you feel full? The power appears to be in their nutritional portfolio. Chia seeds contain 10 grams of dietary fiber per ounce. Fiber takes quite a while to digest and occupies a good amount of space in your digestive tract. Additionally, the 5 grams per serving of protein in the seeds elevates feelings of fullness.

Bottom line — dumping chia seeds in water and slurping it down is not an overnight magic solution to weight loss. But including the seeds in your diet may be a helpful addition to a healthy lifestyle and propel you toward your fat-busting goals.

 Kitchen hacks

Sweet — check. Savory — check. Chia seeds are perfect for all kinds of dishes. Here are some delicious ways to mix them into your meals.

- **Perfect pudding.** Add 1/4 cup of chia seeds to a cup of your favorite milk. Stir well, set in the fridge for at least 15 minutes, and top with your favorite fruit, nuts, or chocolate chips.

- **Dress up dressings.** Give dressings, dips, or sauces a hint of nutty flavor with chia. Allow the seeds time to soak up the dressing and expand before enjoying.

- **Thicken soups and stews.** Sprinkle in a few tablespoons of chia seeds after the dish is cooked.

- **Use a plant-based egg substitute.** If you run out of eggs in the middle of cooking, don't fret. One tablespoon of whole chia seeds mixed in 3 tablespoons of water is equivalent to one whole egg. Let the mixture sit to thicken for about five minutes before using.

Fennel seeds

Can a tiny seed stamp out hot flashes? Details here

Fennel (*Foeniculum vulgare*) is a pretty perennial herb native to the Mediterranean region and in the same family as the carrot. Today, fennel grows in home gardens all over the globe and is even found flourishing in the wild along roadsides. All parts are edible, from the feathery stalks to the delicate yellow flowers and fragrant, lightly sweet licorice-flavored seeds.

Although fennel is well respected for its contribution to the culinary world, its seeds and essential oils offer much medicinal value. One area of study in women's health has turned up some promising results for easing the symptoms of menopause.

From hot flashes to moodiness and insomnia, menopause can be a very challenging time. New research published in *Menopause*, the journal of The North American Menopause Society, found that hormone-mimicking compounds called phytoestrogens found in fennel seeds may make this time of transition less troublesome.

The small study found that taking fennel seed extract for eight weeks improved menopause symptoms compared to a placebo. While you wait on more studies, try these tips to slip more fennel seeds into your meals.

- Add seeds to stew or soup stock.

- Grind them into a powder and use in a homemade salad dressing.

- Mix a spoonful of fennel seeds into muffin or cookie batter.

Flatten a bloated belly and refresh your breath

Move over mints. Fennel seeds are the after-dinner treat you don't want to skip. Restaurants throughout India already recognize fennel's potential and provide a bowl of these seeds after meals. For good reason. They're said to help bust the bloat that often follows eating. Plus they can help freshen your chops.

The tummy benefits are mainly due to the compound anethole, which has a relaxing impact on the smooth muscle of the intestines. That's marvelous for folk suffering from indigestion, gas, bloating, constipation, or even irritable bowel syndrome.

Chewing on fennel seeds offers the additional benefits of banishing bad breath and keeping cavities under control. A study in the *International Journal of Pharmaceutical Sciences and Research* found that chewing fennel seeds increased the pH of saliva and plaque, providing protection from cavities and odor-causing bacteria.

 Kitchen hacks

Are the "munchies" interfering with your weight loss goals? The solution could be as tasty as a cup of fennel tea.

In one small study, overweight women drank tea made from 2 grams of dried fennel seeds before lunch. They reported feeling fuller and ate an average of about 130 fewer calories than those given a placebo tea.

Here's how to make this delicious herbal remedy.

- Place 1 teaspoon of fennel seeds in a mortar, use a pestle and crush until they open and become fragrant.

- Put the seeds in an infuser basket, ball, or bag, and place them in a teacup.

- Boil a cup of water, pour into the teacup, and cover. Steep for 20 minutes.

- Remove the infuser, and add honey or mint to taste.

Flaxseeds

Head off heart disease with less than a teaspoon of this oil daily

Tiny, brown flaxseeds pack a powerful punch. This miracle food contains nutrients that coat your arteries like a nonstick spray, keeping your blood flowing smoothly. That's right, it's an excellent source of omega-3 fatty acids.

These are a good type of fat your body needs, and you have to get them through your diet. Whether you're a vegetarian or just not a fan of fish, a kind of plant-based omega-3 called alpha-linolenic acid (ALA) gives you an alternative to the common seafood sources of omega-3s.

A brand-new study in *Advances in Nutrition* suggests that a small amount of ALA can protect against heart disease — the amount you'll get from just under 1 teaspoon of flaxseed oil a day.

"When people with low levels of omega-3s in their diet ate ALA, they saw a benefit in terms of cardiovascular health," says Jennifer Fleming, an assistant teaching professor of nutrition at Penn State, who worked on the study.

The team's research found that people with high levels of omega-3s from other sources also benefitted when they ate more ALA. The ALA in flaxseeds aids your heart by lowering cholesterol levels and blood pressure, two major risk factors for heart disease.

A few easy ways to add flax to your diet include dropping a tablespoon of flaxseed oil or ground flaxseeds into your morning smoothie or on top of your oatmeal. You can also add them to salad dressings and sauces.

Soothe your skin from the inside out

The origins of your sensitive skin could be a breakdown of the barrier your skin makes between your body and the rest of the world. This would allow irritants to penetrate your skin and cause inflammation.

Fatty acids, like those in flaxseeds, can influence skin health. Research found that eating about half a teaspoon of flaxseed oil a day for three months reduced skin sensitivity and roughness, which are signs of a damaged skin barrier, while also increasing smoothness and hydration.

The seeds have oil in them, too. So you can add them — about 1 1/2 teaspoons of flaxseeds to match the amount in the study — to your meals for a skin safety net.

Fight off joint pain by eating a few of these every day

The creak in your knees, the crick in your neck. These joint pains might be cropping up in your life more than ever. But flaxseeds could be the cheap, easy, and natural remedy you're looking for to relieve joint pain, inflammation, and morning stiffness.

Never swear off these fantastic fats. Osteoarthritis (OA) is a common and costly degenerative joint disease, but current treatments are a bit lackluster at fending off pain and rallying joint function. Experts are looking into other potential healing approaches, and that includes altering your diet. One recommendation is swapping out saturated fatty acids for unsaturated fats, especially polyunsaturated fatty acids (PUFAs), which you can get from flaxseeds.

Some research shows an association between eating more PUFAs and having a reduced risk of worsening OA. In fact, in one study, participants who ate the most polyunsaturated fats were at a 30% lower risk of knee osteoarthritis progression than those who ate the least.

Managing pain with magnesium. This mineral is essential for processes across your body, including bone development, blood pressure control, and muscle and nerve function. Another place magnesium may be key? In your joints.

Research indicates that low levels of magnesium are associated with worse knee pain and function in people with knee osteoarthritis, especially among those who also had low fiber levels. Magnesium plays a role in inflammation, and a deficiency may have an inflammatory effect. This could be why not getting enough of this mineral might be a contributing factor in joint pain.

In one study, over 60% of the men and nearly half of the women with knee osteoarthritis weren't getting the recommended amount of magnesium each day. Men over 50 should get 420 milligrams (mg) of magnesium daily and women should aim for 320 mg. You can get 40 mg of magnesium in just a tablespoon of whole flaxseeds, plus almost 2 grams of fiber.

Lap up the power of lignans

Flaxseeds contain 800 times more lignans than other plant foods. Why should you care? Well, these compounds come with a host of health benefits, and these are just a few.

Extra layer of cancer protection. The anticancer activity of lignans is often attributed to their anti-inflammatory and antioxidant powers. Lignans have another feature, though. One type plentifully found in flaxseeds can be converted into a more active form that's similar to the hormone estradiol. This similarity may give it the upper hand on hormone-related cancers like breast, prostate, and colon cancer.

Boost to brain function and memory. Don't let flaxseeds be a fad food for you. Make eating them a habit, and your brain will thank you. Research shows that feasting on more lignans is associated with less cognitive decline at middle age. That means better brain function, memory, and processing speeds than people who get fewer lignans.

Keep tabs on your weight. Animal studies suggest that lignans play a role in weight control. More human research is needed, but one study found that women with the highest lignan levels had a lower body mass compared to those with the lowest levels. Plus they also gained less weight over time.

So you're ready to load up on lignans, but don't dash off to the store until you read this. Regular ol' flaxseed oil doesn't contain lignans, so you'll need to get your fill from the seeds.

 Boost the benefits

Ready for some fast flax facts? You might think that eating whole flaxseeds is the best way to get this food's nutrients, but that's not the case. Experts think that ground flax may actually be the optimal way.

Whole flaxseeds stay intact as they pass through your digestive system. That means their nutrients aren't absorbed as well. Milling the flax makes good content like minerals and fatty acids easier for your body to absorb.

You can buy flaxseeds that have already been ground, or do it yourself. Storing flaxseeds whole and only milling them right before you use them is actually the best way to keep them fresh with their nutrients intact. Otherwise oxygen can degrade their quality. It's easy to do. Just take the whole seeds you have at home and crunch them up in a spice or coffee grinder.

Pecans

Anti-aging superfoods: 4 reasons to pack your plate with MUFAs

MUFA — sounds like one of those newfangled celebrity baby names that you just don't get, but this is one word you'll grow to appreciate. MUFAs, short for monounsaturated fatty acids, are healthy fats with tremendous health benefits.

Sources of these fabulous, friendly fats include olive oil, almonds, cashews, macadamias, and — you guessed it — pecans. Here's why you should enjoy some of these nuts daily to stay well into your 90s and beyond.

Lessen love handles with a MUFA-rich diet. Studies show that eating a diet high in MUFAs helps keep your belly lean. And a large study of more than 280,000 adults revealed that snacking on nuts is linked to less weight gain and a lower risk of obesity. Researchers say swapping unhealthy foods for a handful of nuts could be a successful strategy to bypass those extra pounds associated with aging.

Choose the fat that keeps your memory sharp. Chewy beef jerky and salty potato chips may be easy to eat on the go, but they have a major downfall. The saturated fat in them is linked to worse brain function and memory. People who eat MUFAs, on the other hand, score better on cognitive tests.

Luckily, pecans are just as easy to snack on when you're in a rush. Plus a study presented at an Experimental Biology conference found that regularly enjoying nuts may strengthen brain waves connected to essential functions such as memory, learning, healing, and cognition.

Munching on pecans is good for your heart. As if you needed another reason to love this nut. In a recent study, people at risk for cardiovascular disease who ate pecans for eight weeks had lower total cholesterol, triglycerides, and "bad" low-density lipoprotein (LDL) cholesterol compared to a control group.

"The addition of pecans to the diet not only produced a greater and more consistent reduction in total cholesterol and LDL compared to many other lifestyle interventions but may also be a more sustainable approach for long-term health," says professor Jamie Cooper, one of the study authors. Even a 1% drop in LDL may be linked to a small decrease in coronary artery disease risk, she says. So the 6% to 9% seen in the study is a big deal.

 Boost the benefits

Light, extreme heat, and oxygen are enemies of healthy fats in pecans, causing them to go rancid and lose their oomph. Use these tips to protect these nuts.

- Store them in the refrigerator for up to six months or in the freezer for up to a year. Use airtight jars for refrigerator storage and plastic zipper bags for the freezer. The great news is that pecans are ready to use directly from the freezer. No thawing time is needed.

- Roasting may improve the flavor of nuts, but does it destroy their antioxidants and healthy fats? Time and temperature are key. High heat and longer roasting times reduce the number of health-promoting antioxidants and break down fats, making them less stable. To reap all of the health benefits from nuts, choose low heat and shorter roasting times.

A small handful of pecans a day could fend off diabetes.
This encouraging information comes from a study published in
the journal *Nutrients*. Researchers from Tufts University found
that just 1 1/2 ounces of pecans daily for four weeks improved
insulin sensitivity in people with excess belly fat. Experts give
MUFAs some of the credit for bringing down your blood sugar.

Easy-to-make pecan salads are bursting with 2 lesser-known minerals

When it comes to inspired pecan desserts, there is no shortage
of options — from pies to ice cream, pralines, and beyond. But
isn't it time you ditch those unhealthy choices in favor of tasty,
wholesome dishes? These pecan salads will tickle your fancy,
especially when you learn they're packed with two trace minerals that often fly under the radar.

Manganese-rich pineapple spinach salad. Trace minerals are
essential nutrients your body needs in small amounts. Don't let
that fool you. They still do big jobs. Manganese, for example, helps
your body break down carbohydrates, absorb calcium, and regulate
blood sugar. You need it for normal brain and nerve function, plus
your body uses it to form connective tissue, bones, and blood clots.

One ounce of pecans — 19 halves — contains 1.3 milligrams
of manganese. That's 56% to 71% of the amount you need
each day. Eat them on a bed of spinach with half a cup of fresh
pineapple chunks to go above and beyond the required daily
amount. To further tantalize your taste buds, top off this
scrumptious salad with tangy feta cheese.

Smashed chickpea and apple salad loaded with copper. This
important trace mineral helps your body absorb iron, form collagen, and make energy. It also maintains nerve cells, keeps your
immune system strong, and assists with red blood cell production.

An ounce of pecans offers 300 micrograms (mcg) of copper and makes a great addition to chickpea salad. That goes a long way toward the 900 mcg you need daily. Chickpeas, apples, and dried cranberries also have copper, giving you an extra boost.

To make a salad, simply rinse and strain a can of chickpeas, and smash with a fork. Then add a diced apple, half a cup of dried cranberries, and an ounce of chopped pecans. Add in your favorite dressing or condiment, and enjoy this on a bed of fresh greens or between whole-grain bread. You'll get all the copper you need in a day in one delicious salad.

 Kitchen hacks

Pecans contain the most antioxidants of any nut — more than almonds and peanuts. So move over almond and peanut butter. There's a new spread in town, and making antioxidant-powered pecan butter has never been easier. Here's how to do it.

- Toast 2 cups of raw pecans on a parchment-lined baking sheet in a 300-degree oven until golden, about 10 minutes.

- Blend them in a food processor on high for a few minutes. Scrape the sides and continue processing until you reach a butter-like consistency. Blend in a dash of sea salt or cinnamon if desired.

- Pour the nut butter into a clean glass jar with a lid. Store in the refrigerator for up to a month.

Enjoy your homemade goodness on whole-grain toast, sliced bananas or apples, celery, and more. Keep in mind, a serving size of nut butter is about 2 tablespoons. Don't overdo it or those extra calories might undo your hard-earned health gains.

Sesame seeds

Beat arthritis pain with seeds of change

Ah — the tiny but versatile sesame seed. You can eat it whole or crushed, raw or roasted, or pressed into an oil. Manufacturers even use it to make soap. But you haven't yet read this surprising use. The seeds may be your answer to nagging joint pain.

That's according to scientists who divided seniors with osteoarthritis-related knee pain into two groups. Both took over-the-counter meds for pain, but only one added a 1/4 cup of sesame seeds to their diet each day. Just two months later the people who ate the sesame seeds reported feeling much less pain than the other group.

That got the researchers wondering why. So they conducted a similar follow-up study and then tested the participants' blood afterwards. They found that the sesame seed eaters experienced decreases in the amount of inflammatory markers in their blood. That's important because inflammation can cause painful and swollen joints.

The researchers aren't exactly sure why the sesame seeds had this effect, but they think it may have something to do with their compounds called sesamin and sesamolin.

So be sure to include sesame seeds in your menu each day. Try sprinkling them into rice bowls, stir-fries, and salads. In addition, they go great over cooked veggies, oatmeal, and yogurt. Or you can try sesame seeds ground into a flavorful paste called tahini, which is used to make hummus. Tahini also makes a tasty salad dressing when mixed with apple cider vinegar, maple syrup, and cold water.

Kitchen hacks

Who knew? Sesame oil comes in two types, each with a distinct flavor and use. The regular version, which is sometimes called refined sesame oil, has a light amber color similar to peanut or vegetable oil. This type is perfect for Asian-style stir-fries because it can withstand high heat. Its slightly nutty taste is relatively neutral and will easily blend into many dishes.

The toasted version, which is a dark brown color, is made from roasted seeds. That gives this oil a much more intense taste. But don't cook with it because it has a low smoke point that causes it to burn quickly. Instead, drizzle the toasted oil over veggies, noodles, soups, or dips. It's also excellent in marinades, and in dressings for cabbage slaw or an Asian-inspired salad. A little of this strongly flavored oil goes a long way, so use it sparingly.

Open sesame! This one-of-a-kind food fights 3 dangerous conditions

Ever hear of oxidative stress? It's pretty much an imbalance between unstable molecules in your body — called free radicals — and your ability to neutralize them. Lots of things can cause this condition, including pollution, smoking, and diets high in sugar, fat, and heavily processed foods.

Over the long term, oxidative stress can damage your cells, tissues, and organs. In fact, it increases your risk of developing high blood pressure, high cholesterol, and type 2 diabetes.

But there's good news, too. You have powerful fighters of oxidative stress right in your very own pantry. Bet you already know what it is — sesame seeds!

Boost your blood flow seed by seed. If you're looking for a slightly nuttier and earthier tasting sesame seed, you'll want to try the black version of this tear-shaped food. But they'll do more than just add flavor to your meals.

In one study, people with elevated blood pressure took black sesame meal capsules daily for a month. The result? Their systolic blood pressure dropped by an average of eight points. Researchers believe these powerful effects come from sesamin, a plant compound found in sesame seeds that is known for its ability to fight oxidative stress.

Keep your ticker in good shape. Animal research has found that sesame oil extracts can lower the risk of atherosclerosis, a dangerous type of cardiovascular disease that can stem from damage to the inner walls of your arteries. Other studies, meanwhile, have reported that substances in sesame seed, namely sesamin and sesamol, work as antioxidants to limit the damage caused by free radicals. This, in turn, allows the lining of the blood vessels to work better.

Has your skin gotten drier with age? Sesame oil to the rescue. It's excellent at soothing and healing, while protecting your skin from UV radiation. Just dab a few drops of refined — not toasted — oil on your face and massage gently until it is absorbed. Your skin will thank you!

Sesame oil helps manage blood sugar. People with type 2 diabetes may want to increase the amount of sesame oil they eat. In a small study, researchers gave folks with this condition either sesame oil, diabetes medication, or both each day for two months.

At the end of that time, those who got both the oil and the medication had the greatest reduction in their fasting blood glucose levels. Here's one possible reason why. The sesame oil increased the amount of free-radical fighting antioxidants in their blood.

Walnuts

A wealth of heart health in 1 mighty nut

What did you toss at the bride and groom after the last wedding you attended? Rice? Birdseed? Maybe rose petals, confetti, or walnuts.

Wait. Walnuts?

If you lived in ancient Rome, walnuts symbolized fertility, and well-wishers commonly pelted the newlyweds with them for luck. Seems a nutty idea today. But walnuts for good health — that is still something to celebrate. Especially since these edible seeds are a good source of B vitamins, several minerals, and — most notably — heart-healthy omega-3 fatty acids.

"Prior studies have shown that nuts in general, and walnuts in particular, are associated with lower rates of heart disease and stroke," says Dr. Emilio Ros, director of the Lipid Clinic at the Endocrinology and Nutrition Service of the Hospital Clinic of Barcelona. "One of the reasons is that they lower LDL cholesterol levels."

That means you should let your heart celebrate with walnuts, because lower cholesterol means healthier arteries, fewer blood clots, and less dangerous inflammation.

Walnuts won't crack under pressure — and neither will you. When cholesterol accumulates in your bloodstream, it can attach to your artery walls, much like grease hardens in your kitchen pipes. This buildup narrows and stiffens your arteries making it much more difficult for your heart to pump blood throughout your body. And that makes your blood pressure numbers skyrocket.

A two-year study on seniors following a traditional Mediterranean Diet had one group supplement with 1 to 2 ounces of walnuts a day while the other ate no walnuts. At the end of the study, systolic blood pressure — which measures the force your heart exerts on artery walls each time it beats — fell by 4.6 points in the walnut eaters. The control group showed little improvement in their numbers.

Through thick and thin, bust up those blood clots. Venous thromboembolism. Deep vein thrombosis. Pulmonary embolism. All tricky phrases to pronounce, but even trickier conditions to survive, since they entail dangerous blood clots.

Too much low-density lipoprotein (LDL) cholesterol in your blood is a known risk factor for these clots. But since walnuts reduce LDL levels, perhaps due to their omega-3 fatty acids, they may also lower your risk of developing these clots.

Ease chronic inflammation with these nuts. A buildup of cholesterol in your arteries can cause your body to go on the offensive, provoking a natural inflammatory response. In turn, this inflammation can cause even more cholesterol to accumulate, and soon you're in a vicious cycle of ongoing inflammation. This can lead to heart attack and stroke. The good news is by reducing cholesterol levels, walnuts can lessen this chronic inflammation.

News in a nutshell: Beat back cancer with this superfood

Eating an ounce of nuts daily is linked to a 15% lower risk of getting cancer, according to an analysis of nine studies. The reason? These tasty treats are loaded with antioxidants, which help repair damage to cells so that they don't mutate into cancerous tumors.

And when it comes to antioxidant powers, walnuts steal the show. Just 25 of them provide the same amount of antioxidants as 8 grams of vitamin C, according to nutrition expert Dr. Michael Greger. That's what you'd find in 100 oranges. Wow!

Read on for two more ways walnuts may help in the battle against cancer.

These tasty tidbits may slow breast cancer growth. The American Cancer Society estimates that 1 in 8 women in the U.S. will be diagnosed with breast cancer in their lifetimes.

Enter walnuts. In a small study, researchers recruited women with breast cancer. Half of them ate 14 walnuts every day for two weeks, while the others didn't. At the end of the study, the scientists found that the tumors of the women who ate the walnuts had genetic changes that could slow their growth.

Women in their late 50s and early 60s who ate at least two servings of walnuts each week were more likely to age with all their mental faculties and without chronic diseases or physical disabilities than women not eating walnuts. Remember a serving is just 1 ounce — or seven whole walnuts.

The scientists believe that compounds in the nuts, including alpha-linolenic acid, melatonin, and vitamin E, may be responsible for the results.

Protect your gut against colon cancer. Colorectal cancer is among the most common forms of cancer in the U.S. In fact, a total of 150,000 new cases of colon or rectal cancer are diagnosed every year. But walnuts may keep this type of cancer at bay.

Research suggests these nuts are great for the trillions of microorganisms, known as the microbiome, that live in your intestinal tract. "Foods like whole walnuts provide a diverse array of substrates — like fatty acids, fiber, and bioactive compounds — for our gut microbiomes to feed on," says study co-author Regina Lamendella, associate professor of biology at Juniata College in Pennsylvania.

Animal studies suggest a healthy gut could hold the key. In fact, they've found that compounds in walnuts enrich healthy gut bacteria, which helps them produce metabolites that offer protection against inflammation and the formation of cancer cells.

Bright idea

Walnuts are loaded with fatty acids, which give them some amazing health benefits. The downside? These nuts tend to spoil quickly. If you have walnuts that smell of old cooking oil, they may not be good to eat anymore. But that doesn't mean you need to chuck them in the trash. Put them to use instead.

Clean up scratches in wooden floors or furniture. Make unsightly nicks or scratches disappear by rubbing a walnut onto them. The oils from the nut will soak into the wood and help cover up the unsightly marks. Make sure to use the meat of the nut and not the shell.

Scare away spiders. Some people swear that leaving whole walnut shells on windowsills or in dark corners of the room helps keep these creepy crawlies away.

Food for vitality — put out the fire of inflammation with walnuts

Munch half a walnut every day and cut your risk of dying from an inflammation-related disease by 50%. That's right — get powerful protection against respiratory conditions like chronic obstructive pulmonary disease (COPD) and asthma, musculoskeletal disorders such as rheumatoid arthritis, digestive ailments like inflammatory bowel disease, and more. All from just half a walnut.

The proof is reported in *The American Journal of Clinical Nutrition*. Researchers followed over 2,500 older adults for 15 years and discovered that those eating as little as 1.4 grams of nuts each day were half as likely to die from a chronic inflammatory disease as those eating less.

To understand how walnuts can help, consider ulcerative colitis (UC), a type of inflammatory bowel disease that affects more than 900,000 Americans. Painful sores in the intestinal walls, abdominal cramps, diarrhea, and bleeding are all symptoms of the chronic inflammation behind UC.

An animal study found that eating walnuts protected colons during UC flare-ups and boosted healing to the tissue lining the colon. Experts believe it may be the omega-3 and omega-6 fatty acids in walnuts, as well as the essential amino acid trypto-phan, that deserve the applause.

And don't forget the profusion of antioxidants in walnuts that can prevent or reduce inflammation throughout your body.

 Kitchen hacks

Put walnut oil on your grocery list if you're looking for a unique flavor that also offers a good-for-you dose of polyunsaturated fatty acids in every spoonful. More great news for your arteries and heart.

Choose a variety that fits your taste and budget.

- **Unrefined cold-pressed.** Generally considered the finest variety, this type is made by pressing ground walnuts until the oil separates from the solids. As the name implies, the oil is not heated. This allows it to keep a more delicate flavor. Best used on cold dishes.

- **Refined.** For this type, a chemical solvent helps extract the oil from the walnuts. Then the oil is heated to remove the solvent. You may notice a slightly bitter taste, but it's fine for sauteing and baking.

Walnut oil may seem like a splurge at the grocery store. But remember, you'll use it sparingly, so the bottle can last a long time. Store it on a shelf where it's cool and dark, and use within six months to a year after opening.

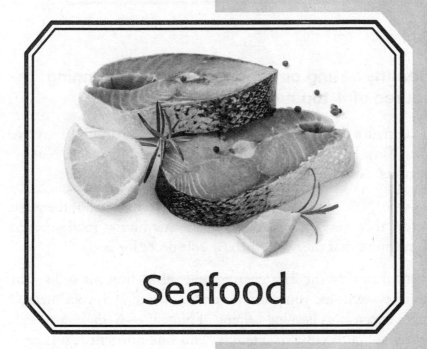

Seafood

Oysters

Healthy eating on the half shell — 1 stunning source of 4 top nutrients

Imagine it's the year 1800 and you're strolling around busy New York City. You pause at a street vendor to buy a snack. Not peanuts. Not a sandwich or even a hot dog. But oysters.

It's true, NYC was once considered the oyster capital of the world. Before they were overfished, these saltwater bivalve mollusks were so plentiful that they were a cheap substitute for beef.

Fast forward to the 21st century and this delicacy is still a nutritional powerhouse you should consider including in your menu. A super reason is its heaping helping of protein — a single raw Pacific oyster contains close to 3 grams. This one nutrient regulates your metabolism and digestion, carries other nutrients throughout your body, and helps your immune system fight infection.

But the good news doesn't stop there. You'll get whopping amounts of these other four nutrients in every briny bite.

Vitamin B12. Think of energy, think B12. This water-soluble vitamin is naturally associated with adding a little more get-up-and-go to your life — especially if you're deficient, as are up to 43% of seniors living on their own. Enough B12 also means your blood and nerve cells stay healthy.

Zinc. Surprise. Oysters are the number one dietary source of zinc. And you'll want plenty of this mineral if you're serious about fighting off bacteria and viruses. At risk of the eye disease age-related macular degeneration (AMD)? Then, again, zinc is your friend. Experts suggest it could prevent damage to your retina and keep early AMD from progressing. Get between 8 and 11 milligrams of zinc every day and your immune system and eyes will thank you.

Selenium. It may not be an element everyone is familiar with, but selenium is vital to a healthy thyroid and necessary for normal cell growth and development. This trace element also protects your body from infection and the kind of cellular damage that occurs during normal aging.

> Oysters have one of the lowest levels of mercury concentration out of almost 70 species of seafood ranked by the U.S. Food and Drug Administration.

Iron. Healthy blood is synonymous with good iron levels and means oxygen from your lungs is carried throughout your body. In addition, you need this mineral to develop nerves properly, create hormones as needed, and even allow your cells to function as they should.

Most oysters sold in the U.S. are either Pacific or eastern oysters, indicating which coast they are harvested from. Experts say the Pacific variety is sweet with a creamy taste, while eastern oysters are saltier and chewier.

Check the following table to see the percent of daily value for these four nutrients in just 3 ounces of oysters. The numbers apply to adults 51 and older.

	Eastern raw	Eastern cooked	Pacific raw	Pacific cooked
Vitamin B12	575	863	567	1021
Zinc	293-403	349-480	128-176	256-353
Selenium	98	120	119	238
Iron	61	83	54	98

Watch out

Correct handling of oysters is vital to your safety and enjoyment. Follow these three rules and you can keep bivalves on your bucket list.

- Purchase oysters only from a reputable seller. If you're in doubt about freshness, ask to see the shellfish harvest tag. By law, retailers and restaurants must keep this on file for 90 days. When stored properly, oysters should be good for up to three weeks from the harvest date listed on the tag.

- Oysters must be alive when you buy them. Look for shells that are closed tightly. Tap two together. You want to hear a high-pitched clank. A dull thud means pass.

- Avoid eating your oysters raw if you have liver disease, diabetes, cancer, stomach disorders, or a weakened immune system. You're more vulnerable to a rare but potentially fatal infection from *Vibrio vulnificus*, a bacteria occurring naturally in coastal waters where oysters live. The good news is thoroughly cooking oysters destroys *V. vulnificus*.

Oysters: Unsung omega-3 heroes defy inflammation

Chronic inflammation is the villain of the century. It's linked to diseases that the World Health Organization (WHO) says are the greatest threat to human health, such as heart disease and arthritis. If that's the battle, then anti-inflammatory foods are your weapons.

While many natural compounds in foods fight inflammation — fiber, phytochemicals like polyphenols and carotenoids, as well as vitamins C and E — omega-3 fatty acids are among the best. They actually trigger what's called an anti-inflammatory response in your body. Just the ammunition you need in this war.

Two specific omega-3 fatty acids, eicosapentaenoic acid (EPA) and docosahexaenoic acid (DHA), are found in seafood, including shellfish like oysters. And scientists have rigorously studied EPA and DHA against inflammation. Here are some important points they've discovered.

- Eat a diet rich in EPA and DHA — fish or shellfish at least once a week — and you're less likely to die of heart disease, compared to people who rarely or never eat seafood. The American Heart Association recommends those with heart disease get about 1 gram per day of EPA plus DHA. Five steamed Pacific oysters contain more than that.

- People suffering from rheumatoid arthritis experienced symptom relief with EPA and DHA. Study participants reported less morning stiffness and joint swelling. Plus they didn't need pain medication as often.

Aw, shucks — 3 oyster myths laid to rest

Who doesn't have a question or two about these interesting mollusks? Maybe you can be the one to drop a pearl of wisdom at your next gathering.

Myth 1. Only eat oysters in the months that end in the letter "r." Perhaps this was true back before refrigeration was widespread, but nowadays, there's no reason you can't enjoy these little gems year-round.

Myth 2. Always store oysters on ice. Yes, these bivalves need to stay cold, but the danger of stashing them in a bowl or bag of ice is that your ice can melt. Oysters immersed in fresh water will die. So tuck them dry in the coldest part of your fridge and cover with a damp towel. Or keep them in a colander over ice.

Myth 3. Swallow raw oysters whole. Connoisseurs insist you'll miss out on that true oyster flavor if you don't give it a couple of chews.

Salmon

Oh buoy! Here's the dish on fish — it staves off stroke

Salmon is one of the most popular fish eaten in the United States. And why not? Its mild taste lends itself to countless recipes. This fish is also one of the healthiest foods you can find.

In fact, you may cut your chance of having a stroke in half simply by eating salmon at least twice a week. That's according to researchers at Harvard Medical School who discovered that women who ate fish between two and four times a week had a 50% lower risk of having a thrombotic stroke than those who ate fish less than once a month.

A thrombotic stroke occurs when a clot blocks an artery supplying blood to the brain. It usually occurs in older adults, especially those with diabetes or high cholesterol and a buildup of plaque in their arteries.

Drab colored food may not seem appealing. But the gray layer of flesh you'll find under the skin of your salmon is better than OK to eat — it's highly nutritious. This fatty deposit is rich in healthful omega-3 fatty acids.

And here's where salmon can help. It turns out that the omega-3 fatty acids in oily fish like salmon, mackerel, anchovies, and herring may reduce the stickiness of platelets, the cells that form blood clots. Moreover, omega-3s reduce inflammation and help relax the inner lining of your blood vessels, an additional aid in keeping clots at bay.

Need another reason to go fishing? A study of more than 1,600 seniors found that those who ate fish at least twice a week were less likely to have signs of blood vessel damage in their brains. That's super important because restricted blood flow to that part of your body — and a subsequent stroke — can lead to dementia, disability, and death. So eat more salmon!

 Boost the benefits

It may be hard not to wrinkle your nose at canned salmon when you can buy fresh. But it's just as healthy as what you'll get at the seafood counter.

Canned and fresh salmon have approximately the same amount of omega-3 fatty acids, but most canned fish offers more calcium. That's because the high-temperature pressure cooking used in the canning process softens the salmon's calcium-rich bones, making them safe to eat.

Another pro is that canned salmon is often wild-caught, and is considered safer when it comes to pesticides than farmed. And like its fresh counterpart, canned salmon is very low in mercury. Plus, it will last on your shelf for several years — no defrosting and cooking necessary.

But if you're watching your sodium levels, read the label for salt content. If there's too much, rinse the fish with water after draining the can.

Blast away bladder blues with this superfood

When you think of vitamin D, your mind probably goes straight to building strong bones. That's one of its key roles, but you may be surprised to hear this nutrient is also essential to maintaining bladder health. Fortunately, salmon is an excellent source of vitamin D.

In fact, a 3-ounce serving of canned sockeye salmon has 17.8 micrograms (mcg) of this vitamin. That's more than the 15 mcg recommended daily for seniors age 70 and younger. And it's just shy of the 20 mcg that folks older than that should get each day.

Here's how this fish helps keep your bladder in tiptop shape.

Urinary tract infections (UTIs). Research shows that women with a vitamin D deficiency are at a greater risk of developing urinary tract infections. Here's a reason why — your immune system needs this important nutrient to fight off infection and inflammation.

Taking vitamin D supplements may be one way to help prevent UTIs. But don't forget about salmon. It's yummy any way you cook it, whether grilled, broiled, baked, poached, or fried.

Urinary incontinence. Ever hear of pelvic floor muscles? They support your pelvic organs, including your bladder, and allow you to control when you urinate. But sometimes these muscles become weak with age. Next thing your know, you're passing urine when you don't want to. Yikes!

But help may be on the way. Scientists found that senior women with high levels of vitamin D were less likely to have problems with their pelvic floor muscles. Makes sense when you consider that you need this nutrient for both muscle strength and neuromuscular function.

Bladder cancer. Vitamin D deficiencies have been linked to an increased risk of bladder cancer. So British researchers worked to find out why. They discovered that the cells that line the bladder activate and respond to vitamin D. This, in turn, can stimulate an immune response.

That's important because the immune system can identify and destroy abnormal cells before they become cancerous.

Great on your plate — a chummy primer on curing

Lox or smoked salmon? When you say one, you may actually mean the other. The key distinction is smoke.

Let's start off with lox. It's a fillet of salmon that has been cured in salt or placed in brine to preserve and season it. Smoked salmon, which is also cured or brined, goes the extra step of being smoked. This adds a woody and smoky flavor to the fish. Lox, on the other hand, has a more salty taste.

Either way, you can't go wrong. When purchasing, be sure to check the label for unwanted additives, place of origin, and an expiration date. Store in your fridge at home, and eat within a couple of days of opening.

Go fish: A handy shopping guide to salmon

Confused between farmed versus wild-caught? Coho and sockeye? And what about mercury content? No need for you to get discouraged — here's the lowdown on salmon.

For starters, farmed salmon are raised in large pens to be sold as food. Wild-caught salmon, on the other hand, grow up and are pulled from their natural habitats.

You can tell the difference between them with a quick glance. Farmed fillets are thicker, have visible lines of fat, and a pale pink color. Wild-caught salmon fillets are thinner and tend to have a deeper, reddish color that they get from eating shrimp and krill. More questions? Then read on.

Which types of salmon are farmed? Atlantic salmon are typically raised this way. Pacific salmon — king, sockeye, chum, pink, and coho — are generally caught in the wild.

Do they have the same nutritional profile? Farmed salmon have more calories and saturated fat than their wild-caught cousins. Both, however, have lots of good-for-you omega-3s and protein, as well as some of the lowest levels of mercury among all seafood.

Which type of fish is more expensive? Wild-caught salmon generally cost more because demand for them often exceeds supply.

Do farmed and wild salmon taste the same? The farmed version tends to have a milder flavor and a more tender texture than the leaner, wild-caught fish.

Kitchen hacks

Sous vide is an intimidating term for a simple process. French for "under vacuum," it's a way of preparing food by sealing it in an airtight container and then cooking it slowly in water at a steady temperature.

Sous vide is an excellent option for salmon — one study found that this method of cooking best protects the healthy omega-3 and omega-6 fatty acids in the fish. Want to give it a shot? You'll need a thermometer and a zip-close bag.

First, place your fish and seasonings together in the bag. Submerge most of the open bag in a container of water, allowing the water pressure to force the air out of it. Seal the bag. Next, heat some water in a big pot to around 120 degrees. Place the zip-close bag in the pot to cook for 40 to 45 minutes. Continuously monitor your water temperature, adjusting the heat to keep it constant. Enjoy!

Quench the fire inside with omega-3s

Chronic inflammation, a condition in which your immune system unnecessarily goes into overdrive, can lead to health problems like rheumatoid arthritis, ulcerative colitis, heart disease, and cancer. So what can you do to fend it off? Eat more salmon.

It's absolutely loaded with omega-3 fatty acids, a family of healthy polyunsaturated fats with anti-inflammatory qualities. Read on to discover how salmon can protect against these other autoimmune-related conditions.

Minimize memory loss. Animal-based research has found that a highly processed diet leads to inflammation in the brain and memory problems. But here's the good news. The scientists also found that supplementing such foods — think deli meats, chips, and frozen pizzas — with a particular omega-3 called DHA reduces theses issues.

Although the DHA in salmon can combat some of the negative effects of unhealthy fare, experts warn that it shouldn't be used as an excuse to eat processed products. After all, such foods are associated with obesity and type 2 diabetes — two conditions you most definitely don't want to get. So why not trade in that greasy drive-thru burger for a freshly grilled salmon fillet?

Fatty fish holds off headaches. Migraines are among the most common causes of chronic pain, with more than 90% of sufferers unable to work or function normally during an attack. Current medical approaches treat migraines with prescription drugs, but what if there were another option?

Researchers gathered 182 adults with frequent migraines and discovered that those who ate a diet high in fatty fish — like salmon — and low in vegetable oil experienced a sharp drop in headache frequency and pain. This study builds on previous, similar research that found omega-3s can reduce the painful inflammation that cause migraines.

Keep vision-stealing macular degeneration at bay. There's strong evidence that inflammation plays a role in the development of age-related macular degeneration (AMD), a condition where you lose central vision because of retina damage.

But the healthy omega-3s in salmon may be able to prevent all that. Australian researchers found that older adults who ate fish at least once a week had a 40% lower chance of developing AMD than those who had it rarely. Even more astounding, those who ate fish three times a week or more slashed their risk by 75%.

The old saying "you are what you eat" applies to salmon, too. And that's creating a difference between farmed and wild-caught salmon. Including more plant-based foods in the diets of farmed salmon is leading to a to a decrease in their omega-3 fatty acids and an increase in their omega-6s.

Wild about salmon? It tops the A-list for B12

When it comes to nutrients, vitamin B12 sure is an important one. You need it to make red blood cells, and it's vital for a healthy brain and nervous system. This vitamin is naturally found in animal products, and salmon is an outstanding source.

In fact, a 3-ounce fillet of cooked, wild-caught Atlantic salmon has 2.6 micrograms (mcg) of B12, more than enough to cover your recommended daily amount of 2.4 mcg. And here's the neat part. Your liver can store this vitamin for a few years, ensuring a steady supply if you're not getting it in your diet.

Unfortunately, though, those reserves can eventually run out. That's particularly dangerous for seniors, because your ability to get enough vitamin B12 from food decreases as you age. One reason why? Older adults are more likely to take medications that interfere with their ability to absorb this nutrient.

If you're wondering if you have a deficiency, be on the lookout for symptoms that include fatigue, palpitations, numbness and tingling in the hands and feet, constipation, a sore tongue, and loss of appetite.

To be on the safe side, talk to your doctor about whether you might benefit from vitamin B12 supplements.

 Kitchen hacks

Try these three tips to improve your salmon skills.

- Drape the fish over an upside-down bowl to help the long and thin pin bones stick out. Carefully run your fingers over the pink flesh, checking for them. Remove the bones with needle-nose pliers.

- Brine your fish to keep it moist and reduce albumin, a protein that congeals into a white goo when heated. First dissolve 5 tablespoons of salt into 5 cups of water. Set your fillets in a pan and cover them with the brine. Soak for 15 minutes, and thoroughly dry the salmon before cooking.

- Have leftovers from yesterday's dinner? Reheat in a way that minimizes the oxidation that creates a fishy smell. Set a wire rack on a rimmed baking sheet. Put the salmon on the rack, cover it with aluminum foil, and place the baking sheet in a preheated 275-degree oven. Let cook until your salmon reaches 130 degrees.

A closer look
Grilling and marinating

Perhaps nothing says summertime quite like a fired-up grill and the savory aroma of sizzling seafood, meats, and veggies in the air. Before you know it, your mouth is watering and the stage is set for a scrumptious meal with family and friends. Doesn't get much better than that!

Oh, but it does. All that deliciousness is guilt-free. After all, when it comes to grilling, there's no sauteing in butter or deep-frying in oil. Nor is anything covered in carb-heavy breading or batter. All that means fewer calories and a trimmer waistline.

Still, you have to be careful. Some studies suggest that charring and grilling meats over high temperatures creates cancer-causing compounds. But don't let that dampen your fun. Just follow these safe-grilling suggestions.

- Clean the grate before placing food on it. This removes any charred buildup from coming into contact with your dinner.

- Cook meats in the microwave for a few minutes before grilling. Doing so limits exposure to dangerous chemicals that may form.

- Trim meat of all visible fat before cooking. Use lean ground beef or turkey for making burgers. This helps prevent lipids from dripping into the fire and producing cancer-causing smoke particles that stick to your steak or burger.

- Grill lots of veggies and fruits. They produce little to no carcinogens when grilled, and this method of cooking enhances their sweetness and gives them a slightly smoky taste.

  Asparagus, corn on the cob, peppers, tomatoes, bananas, and pineapple are all great grilling choices.

- Marinating meats before cooking greatly reduces the number of dangerous compounds that can form. And adding rosemary to the mix appears to make this even more effective.

Speaking of marinades, they add fantastic flavor to all kinds of grilled food — from fish and pork to beef and poultry. Just remember these hot tips.

Homemade is the way to go. Why pay for store-bought marinade when you can easily whip up your own? You'll need just three ingredients — fat, acid, and flavor.

For the first part, go with olive or canola oil. When it comes to acid, choose among vinegar and orange, lemon, or lime juice. You can even use dairy. Plain yogurt, which contains lactic acid, provides an incredible tang that will have you asking for seconds. Use 3 parts oil to 1 part acid.

Now for the fun part. With flavoring, the sky is the limit. Add a touch of salt, garlic, and any chopped herbs you may fancy. Sage, cilantro, mint, oregano, and basil are all winners.

Keep food safety first. Marinate food in a covered glass container or sealed zip-close bag on the bottom shelf of the fridge. This helps prevent bacteria from multiplying and leaks from spilling onto other food.

And never reuse marinade as a sauce on cooked food if it has previously been in contact with raw fish, meat, or poultry. Cross-contamination like that puts you at risk of food poisoning. Yikes!

Time is of the essence. Marinade not only brings out a food's natural flavor. It tenderizes and adds moisture. But leave this liquid gold on too long, and you could find yourself chewing on something akin to dried-out shoe leather.

As a general rule, marinate shellfish, cubed pieces of meat, fish fillets, and tender veggies like eggplant, squash, and cucumbers for 15 to 30 minutes. Chicken breasts, pork chops, and hardy vegetables like onions, Brussels sprouts, and broccoli can steep for a couple of hours.

Save longer marinating sessions of up to six hours for thick-cut steaks and chops, along with roasts and bone-in meats like whole chickens.

Sardines

3 brain-saving reasons you can't afford to miss out on this fantastic fish

Sardines sure don't get the praise they deserve. These surprisingly meaty, slightly salty fish are low in saturated fat and calories, and high in protein. Not only that, sardines are both economical and convenient — lots of people eat them straight from the can.

There's another reason you'll want to add sardines to your menu. They contain three, super good-for-you nutrients that your brain will love.

Protect yourself from just about all forms of dementia with omega-3s. Some 55 million people worldwide live with dementia, and that number is expected to nearly double over the next 20 years. But if you want to lower your chances of cognitive decline, memory loss, and other symptoms of dementia, you can start by simply eating as little as one serving of seafood every week.

In a study conducted by researchers at Rush University Medical Center, scientists tracked the diets and mental health of 915 seniors over five years. The researchers found that those who ate more fish and shellfish had less memory loss and fewer thinking problems. The scientists attribute the results to the omega-3 fatty acids in seafood.

And when it comes to omega-3s, it's pretty hard to beat yummy sardines. They provide more than a gram of these healthy unsaturated fats per 3-ounce serving. That's among the highest levels of any fish!

Pile your plate with sardines to get lots of vitamin D. Your body makes vitamin D when the sun's ultraviolet rays convert a protein in your skin into the active form of this important nutrient. But as you age, it can become more difficult to get regular exposure to the sun. That means you'll want to get extra vitamin D from your food.

And here's why. A study in the *Journal of Clinical Endocrinology and Metabolism* found that the people who got more vitamin D in their diets saw their memory decline more slowly.

> Sardines are a nutrition-packed food that you're probably not eating — but should be. They're loaded with memory-saving vitamin D, heart-healing omega-3s, fatigue-fighting CoQ10, and more. They're no-carb, too!

Once again, sardines step up to the plate. A single 3.75-ounce can of drained Atlantic sardines clocks in at 4.4 micrograms (mcg) of vitamin D. Seniors who are age 70 and under should get 15 mcg of vitamin D every day. Those who are older need 20 mcg.

Selenium helps protect memory. Research has found that selenium may help improve the thinking skills of people with mild cognitive impairment. And now, an animal study may offer some clues as to why.

A team of Australian researchers gave selenium to older mice who showed signs of cognitive decline. They found that this mineral helped improve learning and memory because it stimulated the growth of new neurons in the brain.

Experts recommend getting at least 55 mcg of selenium daily. It may seem hard to believe, but that same 3.75-ounce can of sardines has nearly 49 mcg. Brazil nuts, tuna, and halibut are great sources of selenium, too.

Kitchen hacks

Looking for a new way to enjoy sardines? Try these cooking tips.

Pair them for an Italian treat. Pasta tossed with golden raisins, fennel, breadcrumbs, and sardines is a classic Sicilian recipe. These little fish are great additions to tomato-based sauces, too.

Eat them on top of toast. Sardines make a delicious sandwich if you want a quick lunch or a light dinner. Mix drained sardines with a little bit of lemon juice, olive oil, and fresh, chopped herbs. If you have it, add a bit of thinly sliced green onion before spreading the mixture over toast.

Cook whole sardines on the grill. But first clean and gut them, and then marinate the fish in lemon juice, olive oil, and a healthy pinch of your favorite herbs and spices. If you don't have a grill, you can cook these fish under the broiler, too.

Protect your ticker with some help from this supermarket staple

Just a single serving of sardines a week is a great way to protect your memory and fend off Alzheimer's disease. But why stop there? If you sup on sardines twice a week you can get a whole lot more protection. Experts say these fish are loaded with omega-3 fatty acids that help prevent high blood pressure, stroke, and heart disease. Here's how.

- High blood pressure. This common condition is a major risk factor for cardiovascular disease. And it's often caused by hardening of the arteries, an age-related ailment in which the blood vessels become thick and stiff. Fortunately, scientists believe that the fatty acids found in sardines may help dilate blood vessels and decrease blood pressure.

- Stroke. The Centers for Disease Control estimates that more than 795,000 Americans have a stroke every year. The vast majority of these are ischemic strokes, which occur when blood flow to the brain is blocked by a clot somewhere in a blood vessel. The good news? The omega-3 fatty acids in fish may help reduce this risk. Experts theorize that they keep your platelets from clumping together, allowing your blood to flow freely through your arteries and veins.

- Heart disease. High triglyceride levels and low amounts of HDL (good) cholesterol can create fatty buildups inside your arteries, causing your heart to strain as it pushes blood through them. But research suggests that omega-3 fatty acids lower triglyceride levels while boosting HDL choles-terol, thereby reducing the risk of heart disease.

Want to save global fish stocks? Tap into these wild-caught treats

Raising fish in enclosures to be sold as food uses up a lot of natural resources. For example, a recent study found that it took 515,200 tons of wild-caught fish to produce just 200,480 tons of farmed Atlantic salmon.

What if we simply ate the wild fish instead — especially since they are mostly delicious and highly nutritious sar-dines. Eating wild-caught sardines rather than farmed salmon can help reduce the heavy toll fish farming has on the global seafood supply. And you'll still get all the brain-saving, heart-healthy nutrients you need.

Look for sardines that have been certified sustainable by the Marine Stewardship Council to ensure that they have been caught by environmentally responsible fisheries.

Packed with good health: Eat tasty sardines for peak energy

Feeling tired? You may be tempted to brew a pot of coffee for a caffeine boost. But that won't help you get to the root cause of your lack of energy. If you really want a pick-me-up, snack on some sardines. These fantastic fish are loaded with two nutrients that can boost your stamina.

Fend off fatigue with help from this compound. Coenzyme Q10, better known as CoQ10, is an antioxidant that maintains and energizes your cells. Your body creates it naturally, but the amount you make declines with age. And some medications, like cholesterol-lowering statins, may also cause CoQ10 levels to plummet.

Spanish researchers found that people with chronic fatigue syndrome improved with CoQ10 supplements. And while sardines and other fatty fish are a great natural source of this organic compound, you won't get the amount of CoQ10 used in the study from food alone. So consider talking to your doctor about taking a supplement.

Need more pep in your step? B12 to the rescue. Running low on vitamin B12 is bad news. If your body doesn't get enough, you'll feel tired, forgetful, and foggy. Seniors are more likely to be deficient in this vitamin, so you need to seek out rich sources of it.

That's where sardines come in. A single 3.75-ounce can of drained Atlantic sardines contains a whopping 8.2 micrograms (mcg) of vitamin B12. That's more than three times the recommended daily amount of 2.4 mcg.

The following foods are also excellent sources of this super important nutrient.

- clams, tuna, mackerel, and mussels
- low-fat milk, rice milk, and nonfat yogurt
- beef liver, chicken liver, and ground lean turkey

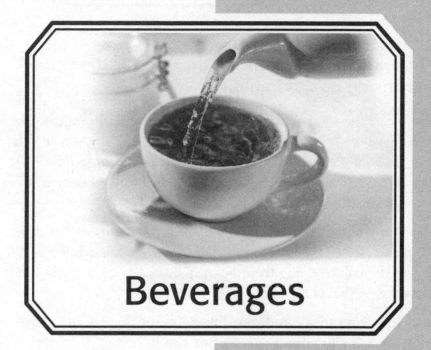

Beverages

Coffee

Grounds for celebration: Drink up for these 2 surprising health benefits

Here's a little-known fact. Coffee gained popularity in the 13 colonies only after the Boston Tea Party in 1773, when switching from "a nice cuppa" felt like the patriotic thing to do. Love for coffee has been growing ever since, and today nearly 65% of American adults drink this beverage daily.

And no wonder — it brings major health benefits to the table. In fact, researchers have found that this everyday drink can lower the risk of dying from heart disease, having a stroke, and developing diabetes.

Sip your way to a healthier ticker. Forget flowers and chocolates, the way to your heart is a hot cup of coffee. A 15-year study of nearly 470,000 seniors — none of whom had signs of heart disease — found that those who drank 1/2 to 3 cups of coffee a day were 21% less likely to have a stroke than those who drank less than that amount. Not only that, their odds of getting a fatal heart disease were 17% lower.

These astonishing findings remained even after the researchers accounted for variables that might impact results, such as smoking status, physical activity, high blood pressure, diabetes, and cholesterol.

"While further studies are needed to explain the underlying mechanisms, the observed benefits might be partly explained by positive alterations in cardiac structure and function," says study author Dr. Judit Simon of the Heart and Vascular Centre at Semmelweis University in Budapest, Hungary.

Raise a cup to fend off type 2 diabetes. You know that eating well and exercising play a big role in staying healthy as you age. It turns out that increasing the amount of coffee you drink can also have big benefits.

That's according to researchers who discovered that drinking coffee — with or without caffeine — can reduce the chances of developing type 2 diabetes. How did the scientists do that?

They noted how much coffee some 120,000 men and women drank each day and then followed their diets. The researchers found that the adults who increased their coffee intake by more than 1 cup a day over a four-year period had an 11% lower risk of having type 2 diabetes than those who made no changes to how much they drank. What's more, those who reduced the amount of coffee they drank raised their chances of getting the disease by 17%.

One of the study's authors, Dr. JoAnn Manson, told Harvard Health Publishing that the chlorogenic acid in coffee — which can delay glucose absorption — may have been responsible for the results.

 Watch out

It's great knowing that the chlorogenic acid in coffee may prevent type 2 diabetes. But another component, caffeine, may be bad for those who already have this condition.

That's according to a small study of adults with type 2 diabetes who experienced a rise in their average blood sugar levels on days that they had caffeine. One possible reason why? The stimulant may trigger the release of adrenaline, the 'fight-or-flight' hormone that can boost sugar levels, says lead study author James Lane, Ph.D.

Further studies are needed to bear out these findings. Still, you may want to switch to decaf if you have type 2 diabetes.

Kitchen hacks

Does drinking coffee make your indigestion flare up? Try cold brewing. Coffee prepared this way is less acidic than traditional hot-brewed coffee, and may be more gentle on your stomach. To make cold-brewed java at home, follow these easy steps.

- Mix 1 cup of coarsely ground coffee beans with 4 cups of water in a large jar. Adjust as needed if you like your coffee weaker or stronger.

- Shake the jar well and store in the refrigerator overnight or up to 24 hours.

- Strain the grounds from the water. Store your cold-brewed coffee in the refrigerator for up to a week.

You can enjoy this drink over ice. Or you can warm it up on the stove or in the microwave. The taste is less bitter, smoother, and is bound to be more gentle on your stomach.

Prevent Alzheimer's disease with a cup of joe

Forgetting your best friend's birthday or where you put your keys is something that happens to a lot people. But as you age, you may start to worry that normal forgetfulness can turn into something much more serious.

Experts estimate that 6 million people in the United States have Alzheimer's disease, a brain condition that impairs memory, thinking, and the ability to do everyday activities. But the good news is that your daily coffee habit could help keep your brain in fighting form for years to come.

In a 21-year study of over 1,400 adults, researchers found that those who drank 3 to 5 cups of this popular beverage a day at midlife were about 65% less likely to develop Alzheimer's or other dementias in their later years.

Why is coffee such a great way to decrease this risk? The scientists aren't exactly sure, but note that the magnesium in coffee increases insulin sensitivity. And that's important because type 2 diabetes can increase the likelihood of developing various forms of dementia.

The researchers also cite the caffeine in coffee. Animal studies have found a link between high caffeine levels in the blood with reduced amounts of beta-amyloids — the proteins that form into sticky plaques in the brains of people with Alzheimer's disease.

That may be why scientists who followed seniors with mild memory and thinking problems found that those with higher levels of caffeine in their systems were less likely to develop dementia than those with lower caffeine levels.

Filter the benefits to beat back Parkinson's disease

Parkinson's disease is a brain disorder that often leads to tremors, stiffness, and difficulty with walking. But it can also cause cognitive decline in its later stages. Fortunately, though, drinking coffee each day just might protect you from this devastating disease.

That's according to researchers in Finland who followed more than 6,700 seniors for 22 years. They found that the men and women who drank the most coffee had a 74% lower risk of getting Parkinson's disease than those who didn't drink any.

Scientists aren't sure why coffee is so protective of the brain. It's thought to be a combination of the nutrients found in your daily brew. For starters, coffee contains lots of polyphenols. These powerful antioxidants may play an important role in the prevention of Parkinson's. While coffee is a great source of polyphenols, you can also increase the amount you get by eating more berries, cocoa, olives, flaxseeds, and nuts.

The caffeine in coffee also appears to play a vital role. An analysis of 13 studies found that this stimulant was linked with a lower risk of healthy people developing Parkinson's. In addition, caffeine has been found to slow the progression of motor symptoms in people with the disease.

While coffee might seem like the go-to caffeine source, here's how other drinks and foods stack up.

- coffee (8 ounces): 95 milligrams

- energy drink (8 ounces): 91 milligrams

- green tea (8 ounces): 28 milligrams

- dark chocolate (1-ounce square): 24 milligrams

Here's to the perks of mood and energy boosts

If you start your morning with a hot cup of coffee — or two — then you know the extra pep in your step it gives you. That's why it's so much easier to tackle your to-do list after you've had some java. And it's not just you who feels that way. Research shows that coffee can keep depression at bay and make people feel more alert.

Improve your mood. We all get blue sometimes, but when it goes beyond the usual sadness, it's time to get help. Sunshine, eating well, talking with friends, and medication can all help to combat and cope with depression. And research suggests that you can add a steaming hot latte to that list, too.

One study of more than 14,400 university graduates found that those who drank at least 4 cups of coffee each day were 63% less likely to be depressed than those who drank less than 1 cup per day.

How does coffee help? It's likely a mixture between caffeine's ability to stimulate the central nervous system along with the anti-inflammatory effect of the polyphenols in coffee beans.

Get energy to do what you love. Do you feel fuzzy in the morning before you've had your coffee? It's a great source of caffeine, which can boost alertness and energy levels. After a cup or two, you'll be ready to take on the day.

Researchers have found that even small to moderate amounts of caffeine can improve the ability to perform a task over a long period of time, as well as improve speed, accuracy, and response times.

But beware, drinking coffee too late in the day can make a good night's sleep hard to come by. That's because caffeine blocks a chemical receptor — called adenosine — that makes you feel sleepy. So if you're having a hard time falling or staying asleep, you might want to cut off your coffee by noon or stick to decaf in the afternoon.

 Boost the benefits

All the sugar and fat in commercial coffee creamers can be harmful to your health. Try the following instead.

- Add 1/4 teaspoon of ground cinnamon, cardamom, or nutmeg to your coffee for a fun, new flavor. Cocoa powder also works well.

- Swap your sweet creamer for coconut milk and a tad of vanilla extract.

- Use a natural sugar alternative such as stevia or monk fruit sweetener.

- Swap heavy cream for skim milk or a plant-based milk such as oat, almond, or soy.

Plant milks

'Moo-ove' over dairy for digestive relief

If a glass of cow's milk leaves you clutching your tummy, it may be time to switch to a healthy alternative that's just as satisfying. After all, plant-based milks provide great nutritional value and are easily broken down in the gastrointestinal tract. Give them a try if you suffer from either of the following conditions.

Lactose intolerance. You're not alone if you have trouble digesting dairy products. Around 30 million American adults have some degree of lactose intolerance by age 20. It occurs in people who lack the enzyme needed to dissolve lactose, the sugar found in dairy products.

This condition leads to uncomfortable stomach troubles, including abdominal bloating and cramping, diarrhea, gas, and nausea, about 30 minutes to 2 hours after eating and drinking foods containing this sugar.

That's why drinking lactose-free plant milks might be right up your alley. Soy and almond milks, for example, are extremely popular. Here's a guide to other types you'll want to try.

- Cashew milk is creamy and sweet like cow's milk.

- Hemp milk provides an earthy, nutty taste.

- Oat milk is thicker and has a sweeter taste than many nondairy milks.

- Flax milk offers a mildly nutty flavor with a silky texture.

- Rice milk has a slightly watery consistency and is a little sweet.

Irritable bowel syndrome. Not all dairy-related tummy troubles are caused by lactose intolerance. Irritable bowel syndrome is a chronic disease that affects the large intestine. The precise cause isn't known, but symptoms often include cramping, bloating, gas, and diarrhea or constipation.

But research suggests that a diet low in carbohydrates known as FODMAPs — short for Fermentable Oligosaccharides, Disaccharides, Monosaccharides, and Polyols — reduces symptoms. One possible reason? The small intestine can have a hard time absorbing these sugar molecules. That leads to an increase of fluid and gas in your bowel and changes the speed in which your food gets digested.

You've probably already guessed that cow's milk is a high-FODMAP drink. That's why if you have irritable bowel syndrome, you may want to switch to low-FODMAP choices like macadamia, quinoa, hemp, and almond milks. Try them all to find which one you prefer the most.

Nutrients — just the facts, ma'am

Plant-based beverages are becoming more and more in demand each day. But their nutrition profiles vary widely, depending on the type of milk and the brand. That's why it's so important to read the nutrition label on the carton before buying.

But here's a breakdown of what you can expect from 1 cup of several types of unsweetened plant milks.

	Calories	Fat (g)	Protein (g)	Carbohydrates (g)
Almond Breeze almond milk	30	2.5	1	1
Planet Oat oat milk	45	0.5	1	8
Pacific Foods hemp milk	60	4.5	3	0
Rice Dream rice milk	70	2.5	0	11
Silk soy milk	80	4.0	7	3

*grams (g)

Heart smart: 2 surprising drinks make a splash

On a mission to keep your heart in fighting form? If so, plant milk could be your new best friend. That's because unlike dairy, most plant-based drinks are free of unhealthy saturated fats linked to high cholesterol levels — a big risk factor for heart disease and stroke.

But the benefits don't stop there. You'll want to drink these two plant milks for their ability to lower your chances of developing coronary problems in the first place.

Drink flax for heart health. You'll definitely want to try flax milk. This creamy, dairy-free option made from blended flaxseeds and water is chock-full of the heart-healthy omega-3 fatty acid called alpha-linolenic acid (ALA).

In fact, a review of studies on flaxseed found that diets enriched with this wonder food can cause total cholesterol levels to drop by as much as 11%. Not only that, the ALA in flaxseeds may protect the heart by reducing inflammation, lowering blood pressure, and preventing blood clots.

Flaxseeds are also incredibly rich in chemical compounds called lignans. Researchers who studied the diets of more than 214,000 men and women found that those who regularly ate foods containing lignans had a significantly lower risk of developing coronary heart disease than those who didn't.

> Before you take the plunge and switch from dairy, remember that not all plant-based milks are free of allergens. So if you're allergic to soy, peas, almonds, cashews, or macadamia nuts, you'll want to steer clear of that particular type of milk.

So load up on flax milk and other lignan-rich plant foods like whole grains, legumes, fruits, and vegetables. Your ticker will thank you.

Sip on soy to lower cholesterol. Soy milk can be a great alternative to dairy as it is packed with protein. In fact, one cup contains 8 grams of cholesterol-busting protein. That's a big chunk of the 46 grams recommended for the average woman and the 56 grams that the average man needs daily.

Researchers looked at over 40 studies and found that, on average, eating 25 grams of soy protein daily over six weeks lowered LDL cholesterol — that's the bad kind — in adults by 3% to 4%. While this might not seem like a lot, lowering LDL cholesterol by just 1% can reduce the risk of a heart attack or stroke.

Dr. David Jenkins, the lead author of the study, says replacing saturated fats and cholesterol-rich meats with soy can spark an even greater reduction in LDL cholesterol. "The existing data and our analysis of it suggest soy protein contributes to heart health," he adds.

Here's another possible way that soy protein helps lower cholesterol levels. It may signal the liver to remove more LDL cholesterol particles from the blood so that they can be converted into bile salts and excreted. Now that's a nifty trick!

No dairy? No problem when it comes to strong bones

A milk mustache could be the key to strong bones as you age, but it doesn't have to come from drinking dairy. Plant milks are fortified with the following vitamins and minerals you need to keep your bones strong and healthy.

Calcium. This is an essential nutrient for bone health throughout your life. Not getting enough calcium can lead to osteoporosis, a condition marked by brittle bones that break easily. Senior men should get 1,000 milligrams of this mineral each day while older women need 1,200 milligrams.

An 8-ounce glass of Silk fortified organic soy milk contains 300 milligrams of calcium. That's 30% of the recommended daily amount for older men and 25% for senior women.

Vitamin D. Getting enough calcium won't do your bones any good if you lack vitamin D. That's because your body can't absorb calcium effectively without it. The two go hand in hand in keeping your bones healthy. In fact, vitamin D deficiency has been associated with a greater incidence of hip fracture in many populations, including postmenopausal women.

Thankfully, several kinds of fortified plant milks provide this essential nutrient. For example, a cup of Almond Breeze original unsweetened almond milk contains 5 micrograms of vitamin D. So drink up — if you're over age 70, that's one-fourth of your recommended daily amount.

Phosphorus. You can't forget to add phosphorus to the list of bone-strengthening nutrients in plant milk. This mineral combines with calcium to form hardened crystals that keep your bones sturdy and rigid.

And you'll want to be sure to get enough. A review of the 2005–2010 National Health and Nutrition Examination Survey found that people who had higher levels of phosphorus in their bodies had a lower risk of developing osteoporosis.

A cup of Oatly original oat milk has a whopping 270 milligrams of phosphorus. That's just under half of the daily recommended amount for seniors requiring just 700 milligrams a day.

 Kitchen hacks

Whether you can't get to the store or you just love experimenting in the kitchen, making homemade almond milk is a breeze. Here's how.

- Soak 1 cup of raw almonds — not the roasted or salted kind — overnight in tap water.

- Rinse the almonds and add them to a blender along with 4 cups of cold water. If you want sweeter milk, add a tablespoon of maple syrup. Blend on high for two minutes until the mixture is creamy and smooth.

- Strain the mixture with a nut milk bag or a couple of layers of cheesecloth. Then pour the liquid into an airtight container. Store your freshly made almond milk in the refrigerator for up to three days.

Shake before using, then enjoy just as you do cow's milk — splashed over cereal, mixed into smoothies, or poured into tea and coffee.

Build your blood with hemp

Getting enough iron sure is vital to your overall health. It's needed for the production of hemoglobin, a protein that enables red blood cells to carry oxygen from your lungs to the rest of your body.

So what happens if you don't get enough of this mineral? You can feel exhausted, weak, and short of breath because your organs and tissues aren't getting the oxygen they need for daily activities.

But hemp milk can help prevent that from happening. An 8-ounce glass of Pacific Foods unsweetened hemp milk provides 2 milligrams of iron — about 25% of the daily recommended amount for seniors.

Of course, you don't want to confuse this beverage, which is made by blending water and the seeds of the hemp plant, with the psychoactive drug marijuana. While they both come from the same *Cannabis sativa* plant, hemp milk doesn't contain any tetrahydrocannabinol, or THC. That's the substance that causes people to feel "high" from marijuana.

Looking to buy hemp milk? Be aware that you might not find it in the dairy section of the market where you'll find, say, almond or soy milk. Most brands of hemp milk come in shelf-stable boxes that don't require refrigeration until opened.

You can make a delicious iron-boosting smoothie by blending a cup of hemp milk with a cup of fresh spinach, five strawberries, and a frozen banana. The vitamin C in the strawberries will help your body absorb more of the iron in the hemp and spinach.

 Watch out

Beware of added sugar in your plant milk. Sweetened versions can have up to 20 grams of sugar per serving mixed in during processing. That's almost 5 teaspoons of the sweet stuff in an 8-ounce glass — more than you'll find in a Twinkie cake. Gee whiz!

The American Heart Association recommends that women restrict their added sugar to around 6 teaspoons per day. For men, that number goes up to 9 teaspoons. Why get so close to your limit with just one serving of sweetened plant milk?

Opt for unsweetened brands instead. Buying flavored plant milks, like vanilla, can help the beverage taste sweeter without any extra sugar. Or you could add 1 teaspoon of vanilla extract to every 4 cups of unflavored plant milk for the same effect.

Don't miss the health benefits of oats

You won't want to shy away from the benefits of oat milk. It's loaded with bone-building calcium. And let's not forget vitamin A, which is so important for eagle-eyed vision. But there's more. Oat milk contains a soluble type of fiber, called beta glucans, that helps prevent digestive issues, inflammation, and dangerous spikes in blood sugar.

Promote gut health and fight inflammation. Who knew that the key to a healthy body is in your digestive tract? That's where trillions upon trillions of bacteria — both good and bad — live. Collectively called the gut microbiota, these bacteria help in the digestion of food and may even influence your mental health.

So, how do beta glucans from oat milk make magic in your gut? The healthy bacteria in your large intestine feast on the carbohydrates they contain, preventing bad bacteria from over-populating your digestive tract and making you sick.

What's more, those sugars later break down into short chain fatty acids that fight inflammation. In its chronic form, inflammation may increase the risk of developing hardened arteries, cancers, and rheumatoid arthritis.

Keep your blood sugar in check. Because the beta glucans in oat milk are soluble, they absorb water to become a gel-like mass that slows digestion. And that's great news when it comes to keeping your blood sugar levels steady.

That's according to scientists who reviewed research on people with type 2 diabetes. They found that eating roughly 6 grams of beta glucans daily over four weeks improved the participants' blood glucose levels.

Along with oat milk, foods rich in this type of fiber include oats, barley, seaweed, and shiitake mushrooms. So drink and eat your fill. Keeping your blood sugar in a healthy range can help prevent diabetes-related complications like cardiovascular disease, nerve damage, and kidney failure.

Skim milk

Blast kidney stones with this beverage

Oh no! Sudden abdominal pain, burning with urination, and even a reddish tint in the toilet. Another kidney stone has come to ruin your day.

If you have frequent kidney stones, you may want to start drinking a glass of skim milk with your meals. A study found that women who ate foods high in calcium were less likely to develop painful kidney stones. And a cup of skim milk has 25% to 30% of your daily value of calcium.

Did your doc tell you to increase your calcium? Then avoid eating high-oxalate foods like chocolate with calcium-rich foods like skim milk. The same process that binds the two compounds in your intestines to help prevent kidney stones also keeps your body from absorbing the calcium.

The reason the mineral helps is pretty simple. The most common type of kidney stone forms when calcium and a compound called oxalate bind together in the urinary tract. When you eat more calcium, it goes to work in your intestines, binding to the oxalates you get from foods such as spinach, nuts, beans, and chocolate. This gets rid of the pair through digestion rather than letting them settle in your urinary tract just waiting to form a stone.

Don't expect the same protection from calcium supplements, though. Researchers think that the difference has to do with timing. People often take supplements without food or with a meal that has little or no oxalates. When you eat them separately, the two nutrients don't have a chance to bind together in the intestines, increasing the chances they'll meet in the kidneys to form a stone.

Got (skim) milk? Drink up for a healthy heart

Country singer Billy Ray Cyrus crooned about his "achy breaky heart" on his debut album. Maybe he should have nursed a glass of ice-cold skim milk instead. This underrated refreshment would have done his heart a world of good. After all, hopping on the nonfat milk train lowers two major risk factors for heart disease.

Sport a milk mustache to banish high blood pressure. Skim milk could be the ticket to steady, normal blood pressure. That's according to Spanish researchers who followed about 6,000 people for two years. They found that two to three servings of low-fat dairy each day — foods like skim milk and yogurt — were enough to cut the risk of developing high blood pressure in half.

What is it about skim milk? Researchers aren't sure, but they think that it could be related to a combination of nutrients. Calcium may play a role by helping blood vessels tighten and relax. The proteins casein and whey may also have blood pressure-lowering effects.

But don't pour a glass of whole milk thinking that will prevent high blood pressure. Even though whole milk has calcium, casein, and whey, it didn't have the same blood pressure-banishing results. Researchers suspect that the high saturated fat content of whole milk could counteract the benefits by reducing the amount of calcium your body absorbs.

Skip the saturated fat for lower cholesterol. The fat debate won't be going anywhere anytime soon. Is it good? Is it bad? Experts just can't seem to agree. But the one thing that hasn't changed is the American Heart Association's (AHA) stance on saturated fat.

The AHA suggests limiting saturated fat to 13 grams per day on a standard 2,000-calorie diet. Skim milk rings in at 0 grams, while two glasses of whole milk will put you over the recommended limit.

Why the cap on saturated fat? This type of fat can raise your LDL cholesterol, forming plaques in arteries and blood vessels and raising the risk for heart disease and stroke.

Milk matchup: 1 carton comes out on top every time

With so many colored caps in the dairy cooler, how do you know which one to choose? Use this lineup based on nutrients per cup to see how skim milk stacks up against the rest.

	Calories	Fat (g)	Protein (g)	Carbohydrates (g)
Skim	83	0.2	8.3	1
1%	102	2.4	8.2	12
2%	122	4.8	8.1	12
Whole	149	7.9	7.7	12

*grams (g)

A 'D'elicious way to get this vital vitamin

Vitamin D is a workhorse of a nutrient. It helps reduce inflammation and supports cell growth, immune function, and the production of energy for your body. If you don't get enough of this fat-soluble vitamin, you're more likely to develop osteoporosis or break a bone.

Vitamin D helps your body absorb calcium, the mineral best known for making bones stronger and less likely to fracture.

Lucky for you, skim milk is usually loaded with both nutrients, so it's the perfect bone-building beverage.

But check the label. Milk isn't naturally high in vitamin D, which means the nutrient must be added during manufacturing. It's not required, though, so you need to make sure you're choosing the right brand. Most skim milks will have about 2.5 micrograms (mcg) of vitamin D per cup, but some offer even more.

That gives you a good head start in reaching the 15 mcg of vitamin D recommended for people under age 70, or 20 mcg for those older. Drinking skim milk along with other vitamin D-rich foods like fatty fish, beef liver, cheese, and fortified cereals and juices can also help you meet your needs.

Switch to low-fat and slow down aging

Skin creams and supplements aside, what if a simple swap could slow down how fast your body ages? Trading out full-fat for skim milk may do just that.

Researchers found that people who drank nonfat or 1% milk experienced several years less biological aging than those who drank 2% or whole milk. In fact, every 1% increase in milk fat led to chromosome changes that translate into an extra four years of cellular aging. Skim milk, with 0% fat, has never looked so good.

Researchers found a stronger association between high-fat milk and more aging when the person's diet was high in saturated fats overall. So pay attention to your whole menu. Besides milk, saturated fat can be found in beef, poultry, pork, butter, cream, cheese, and tropical plant oils like palm and coconut.

While the study can't say for sure that saturated fat or whole milk is a cause of faster aging, the strong relationship is an incentive to swap the creamy stuff for skim or low-fat milk. Making the switch saves you almost 5 grams of saturated fat per cup.

Tea

Brew up 3 piping-hot perks with this miracle drink

What's the second-most-popular drink just after water? Tea, and for good reason. Not only is there a flavor to make every taste bud happy, but this drink is steeped in all kinds of health benefits.

Drink up for weight loss. Eating right and exercising are key to a healthy weight, but sometimes that just doesn't cut it. The Centers for Disease Control and Prevention (CDC) recommends limiting sugar-sweetened beverages to keep your weight in a healthy range. Swap your pop, juice, and sweetened coffee with tea for fun flavor and a smaller waist.

It's not just the replacement effect that helps tea whittle your middle. A large Chinese study found that adults who drank at least 1 cup of tea weekly for six months or more had lower body fat and a smaller waist-to-hip ratio than nondrinkers. Most of the participants in the study drank green or oolong tea.

Researchers think compounds in tea may increase the number of calories you burn and decrease the amount of fat your body absorbs from food. Whatever the reason, adding tea to your weight loss plan can be a tasty way to stay in shape.

Clear your arteries with a cuppa. Want to sip your way to wide-open arteries? Then drink tea. It's one of the best beverages for your blood vessels.

That's according to researchers who discovered that, out of over 5,000 Chinese adults, those who habitually drank tea had healthier and more flexible arteries than those who drank it infrequently. Results were especially positive among people who drank at least 4 cups of tea a day for more than six years. Good news since stiff arteries are linked to high blood pressure and heart complications.

And you won't believe what else tea can do for your heart. A pantry stocked with tea is an easy way to keep your arteries scrubbed clean. Artery-clogging cholesterol won't stand a chance. In a small study, scientists found that 5 cups of black tea a day over three weeks was all it took to reduce total and LDL cholesterol in adults with high levels.

Balance your blood sugar. Just half a cup of cinnamon tea lowered blood sugar after a glucose drink in one small study of healthy people. You can thank the antioxidant-rich polyphenols for cinnamon's powers. Lab studies have found that they have an insulin-like action that could help control blood sugar.

Just don't rely on this kitchen spice to manage your diabetes. The American Diabetes Association says cinnamon isn't a replacement for diabetes medication, but suggests you flavor foods like oatmeal, bread, and smoothies with this warming, fragrant spice to help you cut down on added sugar.

> To brew a mouthwatering mug of cinnamon tea, just use one stick per cup of water and simmer for about 15 minutes. In a pinch, you can mix 1/2 teaspoon of ground cinnamon into a cup of boiling water. Steep for a few minutes, then strain.

Bag the benefits of these herbal teas

Tea enthusiasts may be quick to point out that herbal varieties are not true teas. After all, they don't come from the *Camellia sinensis* shrub, parent plant of black, green, white, and oolong teas. But make no mistake, these blends have tried-and-true health perks.

Rooibos. From the fermented leaves of the *Aspalathus linearis* shrub, rooibos tea has a sweet, delicate, and slightly earthy flavor. It's well known for its bright red color and high antioxidant content. If you struggle with low iron levels, rooibos tea is a great alternative to black and green teas because it doesn't contain any tannins that interfere with iron absorption.

Hibiscus. This tea is sweet and tart, and tastes amazing hot or cold. Instead of leaves, hibiscus tea is made using calyces, the parts of the plant that support the flowers. People in the plant's native regions of North Africa and Southeast Asia have used hibiscus as medicine throughout history. And in one study, researchers found that 3 cups of hibiscus tea daily for six weeks lowered blood pressure in adults with higher-than-normal blood pressure.

Jasmine. Sweet and floral, jasmine petals are often paired with green tea leaves. If you've ever inhaled a fresh cup of jasmine tea, you know how soothing the aroma can be. For some people, just smelling jasmine tea can create a feeling of calmness. However, if you're sipping for serenity before bed, make sure your tea is made with decaf tea leaves.

Kettle kudos: Brittle bones don't stand a chance

Milk gets all the credit when it comes to strong and healthy bones, but the white stuff's not the only drink your skeleton is craving. Add tea to your grocery list to boost your bone health and battle osteoporosis.

While men and women are both at higher risk for developing osteoporosis as they age, women may want to take extra care.

Once ladies hit age 50, they're four times more likely to develop osteoporosis than men.

Surprisingly, teatime may be the easiest — and most elegant — solution. A British study surveyed more than 1,200 women, 65 to 76 years of age, and found that those who drank at least a cup of tea a day had higher bone mineral density than non-tea drinkers. Low bone mineral density can lead to osteoporosis and puts older women at high risk for breaking a bone.

What is it about tea that makes bones strong, especially in older women? Some scientists think it has to do with the isoflavones in tea, chemicals that mimic the bone-protecting hormone estrogen.

 Kitchen hacks

With beads of sweat dripping down your neck, the last thing you want to do is turn the stove on during the hot summer months.

Thankfully, the power of the sun lets you keep your house cool and brew the tastiest batch of iced tea. All you need is a pitcher, water, tea leaves, and a sunny day.

- Add 1/4 cup of tea leaves or dried herbs to a glass pitcher or jar along with 1 quart of water.

- Screw the lid on tightly, give the container a shake, and let it sit in the sunshine for up to four hours.

- Bring the tea inside and strain out the leaves. Add honey to sweeten it if you like, cap the container, and chill it in the refrigerator. Enjoy your sun tea within 24 hours.

Tummy-soothing teas tame 2 major upsets

Feel like you're constantly down and out with tummy trouble? Picking up a tea habit could help banish belly pain caused by everything from inflammatory bowel disease (IBD) to simple indigestion.

The tastiest way to shirk IBD. Stomach pain, bloody stools, and diarrhea. This just sounds like a bad dream for most, but for people with inflammatory bowel disease — chronic inflammation of the digestive tract — it's an ongoing reality. Turns out, drinking tea could provide protection.

Researchers found that drinking a daily cup of tea was linked to a lower risk of developing IBD. How does this work? Scientists think it has to do with the combination of antioxidants and caffeine.

While that's great news for most folks, what if you already have IBD? Well, tea might be helpful, but don't count on it to replace your meds quite yet. An animal study found that green tea extracts act similarly to a popular medication used to manage IBD symptoms. But research is still out on whether green tea and its extracts help people with IBD have fewer episodes.

Pass the peppermint to ease indigestion. Ever wonder why they hand out mints when you leave an all-you-can-eat buffet? It's more than just a tasty parting gift. Peppermint helps calm the muscles in your stomach and makes digesting fat easier on your tummy.

If you feel uncomfortable after a meal, brew a cup of peppermint tea by steeping 1 teaspoon of dried leaves in a cup of boiling water for 10 minutes. Then strain, cool, and sip.

Just be careful. If acid reflux is the source of your belly troubles, peppermint tea won't help and could actually make it worse. While relaxing the stomach muscles helps for indigestion, it also relaxes the valve between your stomach and esophagus, making it easier for stomach acid to rise into your throat.

Watch out

Ugh, a burning stomach and rolling nausea. Did you eat bad sushi last night, or was it something else? It could be the green tea you sipped this morning.

While green tea is known for its plentiful health benefits, it could make you sick to your stomach, especially if your stomach is empty.

Brewing your green tea too hot or drinking it without food in your belly can increase the tannins. These compounds may make your stomach produce more acid, leading to an uneasy nauseated feeling. Keep your tummy settled by brewing your tea after the water has cooled slightly and enjoying it after you've had a bite to eat.

Keep calm with chamomile

Sipping chamomile tea in front of a cozy fire with your nose in a good book sounds like a soothing scene from an old English novel, but there might be something to it.

Chamomile is best known for its calming properties. Does it really work? One of the first human studies found promising results. Chamomile extract reduced anxiety symptoms in people who took 1,500 milligrams (mg) a day over several months. The study didn't use tea, so it's unknown how much you'd have to drink for the same effect.

If anxiety doesn't ail you, but sleepless nights have you dreading bedtime, chamomile tea could be your ticket into dreamland. One study found that 800 mg of chamomile extract daily for four weeks improved sleep quality in people age 60 and up living in nursing homes.

While both studies used extracts, people have enjoyed chamomile as a tea for centuries. It may reduce anxiety and lead to a better night's sleep by binding to the same receptors as benzodiazepines, drugs that are used to reduce anxiety and also cause drowsiness.

Caffeine key — 'pour' over the facts to make smart choices for your health

A caffeine jolt could leave you energized or jittery. While the FDA considers 200 to 300 milligrams (mg) a day to be moderate, this might be too much if you're sensitive to this stimulant.

Unpleasant side effects like nervousness, trouble sleeping, irritability, or headaches could be your sign to cut down on caffeine.

Tea, along with coffee and chocolate, is a natural source of caffeine. Wonder just how much is in your cup of tea? Here's the average caffeine content for 6 ounces of your favorite brew.

	Caffeine (mg)
Black	50
Oolong	30-40
Green	20-30
White	15-20
Herbal	0

With less than half the caffeine as a cup of coffee — which has around 100 mg in a cup — drinking tea can help you cut down your intake without sacrificing flavor.

For some people, though, it's still too much. If you'd love to sip cup after cup of tea but just can't stand the side effects, decaf may be the answer. While herbal teas are naturally caffeine-free, decaf tea has almost all of it removed, so you can enjoy the flavor and health benefits without the jitters.

Water

Tapped out of brain power? Stay hydrated

Water isn't only essential for a strong and healthy body, but also for keeping your brain in tiptop shape.

Even mild dehydration — a condition that occurs when your body loses more fluid than it takes in — can cause cognitive problems like memory loss, confusion, and slow reaction time in making a decision.

It makes sense when you realize that drinking water increases blood flow and oxygen to the brain. Without enough of this fluid, your brain cells can't function properly.

Unfortunately, older folks are especially vulnerable to dehydration. For starters, kidney function can decline with age. This can cause more water to be excreted in urine. And certain medications can increase fluid loss. The good news is that drinking more water can get your brain back on track in no time.

But don't rely on a dry mouth as the sole signal that you're not getting enough liquids. That's because the sensation of thirst gets weaker as you get older. By the time you notice that you're feeling parched, you may already be dehydrated.

So sip on water throughout the day. Drink it at each meal and with snacks, and keep a bottle in an easy-to-reach place. You can also set a timer to remind you when it's time to take a swig or two. And avoid heavily salted foods that can cause your cells to lose water fast.

So, how can you be sure you're drinking enough of this precious liquid? A blood test is the most accurate way to tell, but here are signs that you might be dehydrated.

- headache and dizziness

- dry mouth and loss of appetite

- dark-colored urine

- high heart rate and low blood pressure

- swollen feet and muscle cramps

✗ Kitchen hacks

Boring, tasteless, and bland. If you use these words to describe water, you're probably not getting enough of it.

Thankfully, you can dress up this beverage so that you look forward to drinking it. Fruit, herbs, and vegetables can all infuse your water with fresh and tasty flavor combinations.

You could use a special pitcher outfitted with a basket to hold the ingredients you wish to steep. But it really isn't necessary.

Simply place the delicious additives in a glass jar. Fill it with cold water and let the jar sit in the refrigerator for a few hours or overnight. Strain the contents before pouring in a glass. Drink within a couple of days.

Fun flavor combinations include sliced cucumber, mint sprigs, and chunks of honeydew melon. You could also mix strawberries, basil, and lemon slices in your water. The sky's the limit when it comes to making your own.

Skipping stones: Filter your body sip by sip

Bet you can't guess what Michelangelo, Alfred Hitchcock, and the singer Billy Joel had in common. Give up? Aside from being famous in their careers, all three suffered from kidney stones — pebble-like pieces of minerals that can form inside your kidneys.

And boy, they sure can be painful. That's why it's so important to drink your fill of water. Doing so dilutes your urine and helps prevent these stone-forming crystals from sticking together.

So how much should you drink? A review of studies on the subject found that people who drank at least 8 1/2 cups of water daily had a nearly 10% lower risk of developing a kidney stone than those who drank around 6 cups a day. Those odds improved even further among folks who drank 13 cups per day.

So be sure to get enough water, particularly during the hot summer months. Losing water through sweat leads to reduced urine production. And the less you urinate, the more likely your chances of having minerals settle and bind together in your kidneys.

The most common kidney stone is made of calcium and oxalate. But you can still enjoy calcium-rich dairy and leafy greens as well as high-oxalate fare like beets and peanuts. The secret? Eat these types of foods together so that the compounds bind in your gut instead of your kidneys.

Raise a glass to the pursuit of wellness

Drinking water is the single most important thing you can do to maintain healthy skin, hair, and nails. Not only that, this naturally fresh beverage is essential to keeping your internal body functions running smoothly. Here's how.

Regulates body temperature. You might be surprised to learn that water accounts for roughly 60% of an adult's weight. All that liquid helps transport nutrients and oxygen to your cells. Moreover, it acts as a built-in air conditioner.

How's that? Let's say you're gardening under the hot sun. Next thing you know, you begin to sweat. No worries, it's your body's way of cooling itself. As the water evaporates from your pores into the air, it cools the area around your skin and makes you feel more comfortable. Pretty neat trick.

Of course, you'll want to replace all that water lost through perspiration. Otherwise, you might become dehydrated. That can lead to all sorts of problems, including weakness, dizziness, and confusion.

So how much water should you drink if you find yourself sweating heavily? While there's no one-size-fits-all answer, as a general rule healthy adults should aim for at least two to three glasses per hour.

Keeps blood pressure and heart rate stable. Dehydration can cause your blood volume — the amount of fluid in your blood vessels — to drop dramatically. Soon after, your blood pressure takes a nosedive and your heart begins to work extra hard, pumping faster and faster to keep your blood moving. Not good.

Oddly enough, that same lack of water could also send your blood pressure through the roof. When you're dehydrated, your brain sends a signal to the pituitary gland to release vasopressin — a hormone that causes your blood vessels to constrict. This can spark a rise in blood pressure.

The simple solution for both problems? Drink lots of fluids. The recommended amount for men is 15 1/2 cups a day. Women should have 11 1/2 cups daily. That includes all beverages, and even fruits and veggies. Cucumbers, celery, tomatoes, cantaloupe, and strawberries all contain lots of water.

And while all fluids help to hydrate you, some are healthier than others. So stay away from sugary drinks and opt for water, the low-cost and no-calorie winner.

Fussing with filters — think before you drink

Funky flavors or odors may indicate that harmful chemicals are lurking in your tap water. But how do you know which ones they might be?

If you're on municipal water and pay your own bill, you should receive an annual water quality review called a Consumer Confidence Report. If you rent, contact your landlord to get the ball rolling. Utilities that provide water to more than 100,000 people have to post such information online.

If you use well water, the Environmental Protection Agency recommends getting your water tested at a certified lab. Go to *epa.gov/ground-water-and-drinking-water* for more information.

Once you learn if your water is contaminated — chemicals can include arsenic and lead — you can buy the proper type of filtration system. Just be sure to purchase one that's approved by NSF International and the American National Standards Institute.

Simple ways to get going when you're backed up

Ugh, constipation. It's a common gastrointestinal problem marked by bowel movements that are infrequent or difficult to pass. And although it's rarely talked about, this condition affects more than a third of adults over age 60. If you're one of them, drinking extra water can help.

That's because skimping on this life-giving beverage makes you dehydrated. When that happens, your body is forced to draw water from the large intestine. The result? Hard, dry, and lumpy feces that are painful to excrete.

Now you've probably heard that one of the easiest ways to remedy constipation is to eat more fiber. While that's true — senior women and men should get 21 and 30 grams daily, respectively, from whole grains, fruits, legumes, and veggies — water helps all that fiber bulk up your stool so that it is more quickly and easily eliminated.

Researchers tested this when they separated folks with constipation into two groups. Both of them ate 25 grams of fiber daily over two months. But the participants who drank around 8 1/2 cups of mineral water each day experienced a bigger increase in the frequency of bowel movements than those who drank a little more than 4 cups of liquid each day. They were also less reliant on laxatives.

Joint resolution: Get a grip on pain

Did you know that drinking a glass of refreshing water can take the edge off your arthritis pain and ease a world of other hurts? Read on to find out how.

Drink up for relief. You're not alone if arthritis keeps you from doing the things you love. Nearly half of all U.S. seniors over 65 have been diagnosed with the disease. But treating yourself with water can help eliminate the pain and keep you moving by ensuring there is enough cushion around your joints.

That's because water is an essential part of a thick liquid called synovial fluid that lubricates your joints and keeps them operating smoothly. Dehydration can make it hard for your body to produce this fluid, leading to increased friction and pain when you move.

But it's not just synovial fluid that keeps your joints working like a well-oiled machine. It's estimated that up to 80% of cartilage, the spongy material that allows your bones to seamlessly glide over each other when flexing and straightening your joints, is made of water. If you don't drink enough of this beverage, your cartilage can become stiff and dry. And that can lead to inflammation of the joint. So stay hydrated.

Say goodbye to gout. If you've ever had a gout attack, you know how excruciating the pain can be. This type of arthritis is caused by eating foods high in purines — compounds that break down into uric acid in your blood — that cause painful crystals to build up in your joints. The end result? Severe swelling, redness, and tenderness in the affected area, usually the big toe.

Thankfully, there's an easy way to decrease the frequency and severity of gout attacks. The Arthritis Foundation recommends drinking eight glasses of water a day to help prevent a gout attack and up to 16 glasses during a flare-up. All that water will help flush the uric acid from your system.

> You may want to limit or avoid certain fare if you suffer from gout. Foods high in purines — including red and organ meats, anchovies, trout, scallops, sardines, tuna, and drinks sweetened with fructose — can lead to a flare-up.

Tame your aching head with this thirst quencher

If you're one of the 15% of American adults who complain of severe headaches or migraines, you know how easily they can knock you down. But what if instead of reaching for painkillers you could ease the throbbing with a tall glass of refreshing water?

You've probably already guessed that dehydration can trigger an aching head. It makes sense considering that a lack of water can cause your brain to contract and pull back from your skull. Next thing you know, you're in a world of hurt.

Here's how to know if a lack of fluids may be causing your headache. The pain, which can range from dull to severe, generally appears on the front, sides, or back of your head. Bending over, shaking your head, or moving around can make it feel worse.

But it's unlikely that you'll feel pressure on your face. That type of pain often comes with a sinus headache. Nor will you probably experience discomfort at the back of your neck brought on by too much tension.

If you think you have a dehydration headache, take slow and steady sips from a glass of water or two as soon as you can. The pain should disappear within a few hours.

 Bright idea

Tired of bubbling water rising to the point of boiling over whenever you cook pasta? Place a wooden spoon lengthwise over the diameter of your pot. It will stop any overflow from splashing onto your stovetop.

Of course, after your noodles are al dente, you'll want to save some of the cloudy water left behind. It's like liquid gold because pasta releases starch — a type of carbohydrate found in grains and other foods — into the liquid while it simmers.

Adding a little of this starchy goodness helps other ingredients — say olive oil, herbs, garlic, and shredded parmesan cheese — stick to your noodles. It also thickens any sauce you're making, giving it a silky texture. And don't be afraid to save your pasta water for future recipes. Freeze it in an ice cube tray and add a cube or two to soups, stews, gravies, or even risotto. Bon appétit!

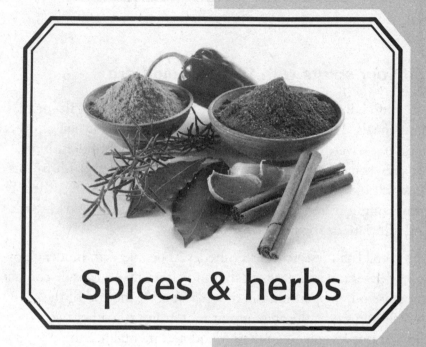

Spices & herbs

Anise

Lift your spirits with this age-old herb

Ancient civilizations used anise seeds to add a pop of flavor to their meals. They also believed that these tiny treats had another benefit — warding away dark thoughts and nightmares. Now, modern scientists think there may have been some truth to this superstition. While these seeds won't relieve nightmares, there is promising research to suggest they can improve people's moods and alleviate depression symptoms.

In a small trial, researchers recruited 120 people with moderate or mild depression and assigned them to either take a capsule containing anise oil, peppermint oil, or a placebo. At the end of the monthlong study, the anise group — but not the other two — showed improvements in their mood and mental health.

More research needs to be done to understand exactly how this herb can fend off depression. If you're interested in trying it yourself, people in the study took three capsules containing 200 milligrams of anise oil every day. You can find this supplement online or in local grocery stores. However, if you have diabetes or estrogen-sensitive cancer, talk with your doctor before taking anise. It may cause dangerous interactions with your medications.

Bye-bye bloating: Get natural relief from digestive woes

Even though many herbal remedies are based on folklore, the oils or seeds from some herbs are better at relieving gas than many commercial products.

For instance, cakes flavored with anise were popular in Roman times to prevent indigestion after a particularly rich meal, such as a wedding feast. And by the way, this is where the tradition of a wedding cake came from. Brilliant, right?

Today, crush 1 1/2 teaspoons of anise seeds with a mortar and pestle. Bring 1 cup of water to a boil. Turn off the heat, and add your spice. Let steep for 10 to 15 minutes, then strain and drink it hot to relieve gas pain.

Interested in other herbs to deflate your gas? Give one of these a try.

- Tea made from chamomile is an old and familiar prescription for calming and healing the digestive system.

- Peppermint leaves, either chewed or steeped in hot water, can relieve gas and indigestion.

- Fennel was once used as a guard against witches, fleas, and bad spirits — quite a burden of responsibility for such a delicate looking herb. Crushed fennel seeds, mixed with anise and caraway, make a soothing tea.

- The seeds of the caraway plant add flavor and reduce the gassy side effects of foods like cabbage.

 Watch out

Star anise and anise seeds may have a similar name and flavor, but these two plants come from completely different families. If you're after anise's health benefits, don't mix them up.

- Anise seed (*Pimpinella anisum*). This tiny herb is related to dill, cumin, and caraway. It has a slightly spicy, licorice-like flavor that's often used to flavor Mediterranean baked goods and sausages.

- Star anise (*Illicium verum*). This star-shaped pod is a part of many Asian spice blends, and its flavor is a bit stronger than anise seeds. The pod is added to stews and soups to add spice and sweetness.

Cinnamon

3 reasons to sprinkle on this heartwarming spice

Experts estimate that heart disease is responsible for 25% of all deaths in the United States. The good news? A dash of cinnamon could help you avoid suffering from some of the major risk factors, like high cholesterol, high blood pressure, and obesity.

Curb your cholesterol with a little bit of cinnamon. Think of your veins and arteries as if they're highways for your blood cells. If they're smooth, clean, and clear then it's easy for your heart to pump blood where it needs to go. But if you have too much cholesterol in your body, this waxy, sticky substance can create traffic jams that slow down the blood flow and make your heart work overtime to keep everything moving.

Fortunately, cinnamon may help bust up those traffic jams. An analysis of 13 studies found that cinnamon lowered total cholesterol levels. More research is needed to nail down just how much cinnamon you need to take, and for how long, but in the meantime you can use this spice to add flavor to your meals in place of sugar or fat.

Lower blood pressure with help from this sweet spice. A new study revealed that cinnamon may be a great way to bring high blood pressure down. Researchers recruited people with hypertension, and assigned them to one of two groups. Half of the people received a placebo, while the others got a capsule loaded with cinnamon.

After three months, the people who took cinnamon had lower systolic blood pressure. The reason? Experts think naturally occurring compounds in cinnamon called phytochemicals help the blood vessels relax, which lets blood flow through more easily.

The volunteers in this study who took cinnamon received a capsule containing 1,500 milligrams, which is a little bit more than a half a teaspoon.

Add a dash of cinnamon to trim your waistline. Carrying around a few extra pounds? You're not alone. The Centers for Disease Control and Prevention estimates that nearly 3 out of every 4 Americans are overweight. While this condition may be common, it's bad news for your heart health. Excess weight increases your risk of heart disease, high blood pressure, and other potentially life-threatening conditions.

Your spice cabinet may have a secret ingredient to help you slim down. In a small study, researchers recruited 116 volunteers with metabolic syndrome and asked them to either take a capsule containing wheat flour or 1 1/2 teaspoons of cinnamon. After four months, the cinnamon group dropped more weight than those who took the flour capsules.

Sweet solution for tummy troubles

Cinnamon isn't just for sweet buns. In traditional Greek and Indian medicine, cinnamon treats bloating, indigestion, nausea, gas, and gastrointestinal spasms. Its healing capabilities and sweet taste have made it a valuable spice for thousands of years.

Powerful defense against food poisoning. Cinnamon spice is nice, except to bacteria, like *E. coli*, a dangerous bacterium that causes severe diarrhea and flu-like symptoms. It usually turns up in unpasteurized food and undercooked meat.

But the bark, leaves, and roots of the cinnamon tree all produce essential oils containing a substance that kills germs, especially *E. coli*. The proof? Researchers added cinnamon to apple juice infected with a large sample of *E. coli*. After three days at room temperature, the cinnamon destroyed more than 99% of the bacteria.

Find comfort from upset stomach. Adding cinnamon to your meal does more than kill bacteria. The volatile oils break down fats in your intestinal tract, and the essential oils stimulate movement. This double action gets your system back to normal and relieves that bloated feeling.

It also aids digestion, even though scientists don't know exactly what cinnamon does to help. It may have something to do with the way the spice heats up your stomach.

 Bright idea

Found a tin of cinnamon that's been hiding in your pantry for years? It's probably past its prime. Ground spices lose their flavor and potency after about six months. But you don't need to toss them. You can still use them around your house, and save yourself a few bucks while you're at it.

- Use cinnamon to keep pests away. Sprinkling cinnamon around doorways or windowsills may prevent ants and silverfish from finding their way into your house.

- Soothe bug bites with a cinnamon salve. Mix together a tablespoon of honey and cinnamon, and spread it on a mosquito bite to help with the itchiness.

- Mix expired cinnamon or other sweet-smelling spices with baking soda and sprinkle it on your carpet. Let it sit for a few minutes and then vacuum it up to release the essential oils into the air.

Cinnamon tea gets your gut back on track

The spicy aroma and flavor of cinnamon may make it one of the most beloved condiments in your kitchen. It's versatile enough to pep up a sweet dish or add a subtle warmth to stews and curries. But as popular as it is for cooking, cinnamon has an even longer history in folk medicine. From ancient Egypt and China to Europe in the Middle Ages, herbalists used cinnamon against a slew of digestive ailments. Today, you can whip up your own home remedy in no time.

Start with 4 cups of boiling water. Add 1/4 teaspoon of cayenne pepper and 1/2 teaspoon of cinnamon. Simmer your tea for five minutes. Remove from heat and steep for 10 minutes. For flavorful relief from diarrhea, drink 1/4 cup every half hour.

Another delicious tea, popular with the Pennsylvania Dutch, combines 1/8 teaspoon of cinnamon, 1 teaspoon of nutmeg, and a little honey in a cup of warm milk. Drink at mealtime to soothe symptoms of diarrhea. For a little extra zing, add a pinch of powdered cloves, like they do in Brazil.

 Watch out

For some sensitive people, cinnamon is one of the worst culprits when it comes to causing canker sores. You may have already dropped red-hot candies, cinnamon-flavored chewing gum, and cinnamon buns. But it also hides in foods like cookies, cereals, and chili recipes, or flavored drinks. And it's sometimes added to mouthwashes, toothpastes, and breath fresheners to make them taste better.

Canker sores usually appear in places that come in direct contact with the cinnamon. People who frequently suck on hard candies tend to get them on one side of the tongue or cheek. Cinnamon tea drinkers, on the other hand, are more likely to get them throughout the mouth.

To avoid an unpleasant surprise, it's a good idea to check the label for this hot ingredient in any product you put in your mouth.

Cloves

Want to curb high blood sugar? Favor these fragrant buds

About 1 out of every 10 Americans has diabetes. Most of them have type 2 diabetes, which means their cells don't respond normally to insulin, a hormone the body needs to break down and use sugars. If it's not properly managed, this condition can damage your nerves and kidneys, and even lead to stroke and heart disease.

Diabetes doesn't set in overnight, though. Before most people develop this condition, they get something called prediabetes. Their cells become resistant to insulin, so they have chronically high blood sugar. But there's still time to reverse the damage.

If you have prediabetes, you may want to look to your spice rack for a bit of help. Cloves — those pungent flower buds used to flavor meat, sauces, desserts, drinks, and rice dishes — have a hidden talent. A small, preliminary study found that clove extract can bring down people's blood sugar. The results came after researchers gave volunteers with prediabetes 250 milligrams of clove extract for 30 days.

Save your furniture and your sanity by rubbing a little oil of cloves onto wooden furniture items — not fabric — that your puppy is chewing. He won't like the smell or the taste.

You can find clove extracts online or at some health food stores. However, before you start taking these supplements, talk to your doctor about any conditions or medications you're on. Cloves may cause dangerous interactions with certain prescriptions, such as blood thinners or diabetes medication.

Kitchen hacks

Cloves are actually the dried, unopened flower buds of a tropical evergreen tree native to the Spice Islands of Indonesia. They are pink or green when harvested, then turn a dark brown as they dry. The word cloves comes from the Latin *clavus*, which means nail. If you look at a clove closely, you'll see it resembles a tiny nail, a shape that comes in handy when using cloves to stud oranges or a ham.

Although you can buy ground cloves, try grinding your own to retain more of the essential oils.

- Use a granite mortar and pestle to powderize whole cloves. Work in small batches, and use a twisting motion with your pestle for best results.

- Crush your cloves in a metal spice grinder. Never use one with plastic parts since the clove oils will degrade and cloud the plastic.

Experts also suggest using a small food processor, a blender, or a clean pepper mill.

Tooth wisdom: Soothing oil stops cavity agony

Think cavities are just for kids? Not true. More than 90% of adults over age 40 have had at least one cavity. And conditions associated with aging — such as dry mouth or gum disease — can increase your risk.

Usually, tooth decay doesn't cause discomfort. But if bacteria and plaque eat through the protective enamel on your pearly whites and reach the nerve, that cavity can cause your teeth to hurt. Contact a dentist as soon as you can if you have a toothache. But while you wait to get the tooth checked out, you can tame the pain with a dab of clove oil.

In a small study, researchers found that clove oil was just as effective at numbing the mouth as a traditional over-the-counter anesthetic gel. Want to give it a go? Simply soak a cotton swab in the essential oil and hold it on your sore tooth for about 10 seconds. Avoid swallowing any of it.

Bright idea

Mothballs may protect your clothes from destructive moths, but what will protect your clothes — and you — from the unpleasant smell of mothballs? Try this spicy, sweet alternative — whole cloves. Bugs hate them just as much as mothballs.

Simply put some cloves in cheesecloth or a small muslin drawstring bag. It's an ingenious way to repel bugs and freshen clothing. Tuck your clove sachet into a drawer or closet. No more mothball odor.

You can also just put a few individual cloves in the pockets of your wool coats, jackets, and hats.

3 creative ways to spice up your home

Can't get enough of the warm, woodsy scent of fresh cloves? This spice is good for more than adding that little bit of sweet heat to holiday recipes and mulled cider. Here are some ways to use it around your house year-round.

- Whip up a simple air freshener by adding a few drops of clove essential oils to a spray bottle. Top it off with water and spritz it throughout your house.

- Cover up cooking smells with whole cloves. Simmer a few cups of water in a small pan and add a smatter of whole cloves to the water. In a matter of minutes, your kitchen will smell sweet and spicy.

- Wipe out messes with a homemade cleaning solution. Mix 1/2 teaspoon of clove oil with 1 1/2 cups of warm water, and use it to scrub away foul-smelling molds and mildew.

A closer look
Low-salt diet

Hard to believe, but salt was once so valuable that Roman soldiers were sometimes paid with this seasoning instead of money. Nowadays it's easy to get your hands on salt — maybe too easy.

The average American eats nearly 3,400 milligrams of sodium every day. That's well over the daily limit of 2,300 milligrams — equal to a mere 1 teaspoon of table salt — that experts recommend for healthy adults. This salt overload spells bad news. High-salt diets have been linked with an increased risk of heart problems, high blood pressure, stroke, kidney disease, and even stomach cancer.

Fortunately, with a little know-how you can lower your salt intake without sacrificing flavor.

Cut down on hidden sources of sodium. Setting down the salt shaker is a fantastic start when you're trying to prune out sodium, but the bulk of your daily salt intake isn't coming from table salt. Prepackaged and processed foods, like canned soups and veggies, deli meats, and jarred sauces are often loaded with salt.

One of the best ways to slash salt is to opt for fresh fruits, veggies, and meats whenever possible. If you do buy canned or packaged foods, look for ones labeled "low sodium" or "no salt added." Avoid prepared meals that contain more than 600 milligrams of sodium. You can also talk to your grocery store and see if they can recommend low-sodium products.

If you have canned veggies or beans in your pantry, you don't need to throw them out just because they're high in salt. Experts at the USDA estimate that draining and rinsing canned goods can remove up to 23% of the salt content.

Are low-sodium substitutes worth their salt? If you're following a low-sodium diet, you may be intrigued by the salt substitutes on the shelf of your local grocery store. But will these alternative options really fill the salt-shaped hole in your flavor palate?

- Potassium chloride. These salt substitutes look like salt and have a bit of a salty flavor, but they don't have any sodium. Some people also think they have a bitter, metallic taste.

  If you take certain medications, the high levels of potassium may cause dangerous interactions. Talk to your doctor if you're considering a potassium-based salt substitute.

- Low-sodium salt. Some companies make a salt substitute that's part table salt and part potassium chloride. The result is a salty, tasty seasoning with often half the sodium levels of regular salt. It still contains a fair amount of sodium, though, so you should use it sparingly.

- Nutritional yeast. This savory and nutty seasoning doesn't taste particularly salty, but it adds a flavorful punch. It's also loaded with B vitamins, is low in fat and sodium, and offers up a healthy amount of zinc, fiber, and protein.

  Many people love nutritional yeast on popcorn, eggs, and even sprinkled over roasted veggies. It also goes great in pasta and rice dishes, and makes a delicious topping on roasted chickpeas.

Amp up flavor without reaching for the salt shaker. Herbs and spices are a great way to impart flavor without piling on sodium. However, if your dishes are still missing a little something, punch up your meals with these salt-free hacks.

Add a splash of acid to your meal. A little bit of vinegar or a spritz of citrus juice can help lift the natural flavors of food and add brightness to your dish. Experiment with different types of vinegar or citrus to see which pairs best with your dinner.

Let your food cool some before you adjust the seasoning. Your food may taste a little bland when it's piping hot, only to taste too sour, spicy, or salty by the time it hits the dinner table. The reason? The receptors on your tongue are less sensitive to very hot — or very cold — foods.

Ginseng

Herbal help for colds and flu

Get a little boost during cold and flu season with a ginseng supplement. This popular herb has been used in traditional Chinese
medicine for more than 2,000 years to increase strength and energy,
while reducing stress and fatigue. It can give you a stronger
immune system by working in several surprising ways.

- triggering your body to produce more T cells, a type of white
  blood cell that seeks out and destroys bacteria and viruses
- adding extra power to any antibiotics you might be taking
  for a bacterial infection
- giving your flu shot a little added oomph

Many people swear their daily dose of ginseng means shorter
and fewer colds than usual.

The ginsenosides in ginseng also give the herb some antioxidant
power, making it useful in the fight against high cholesterol,
memory loss, high blood pressure, and many other conditions
where dangerous free radicals cause damage.

A botanical to battle stress

Stress is as old as the ancient struggle for life, and as modern as
your busy schedule. But ginseng is a remedy that has been passed
down through the years. It's known as an adaptogen, or a treatment that works in a nonspecific way to cut stress without doing
your body any harm.

Some researchers think ginseng stops stress by indirectly recharg-
ing rundown adrenal glands, which help your body react and

adapt in times of stress. When constant stress has left your adrenals run down and worn out, ginseng gets them going again. Once the adrenals are recharged, they can continue to help your body rebound from stress.

Active ingredients in ginseng are called ginsenosides, a type of natural plant chemical. You'll find several types of ginseng available, including American ginseng, Chinese or Korean ginseng, and Siberian ginseng. Experts suggest you look for a product labeled *Panax ginseng* that has been standardized to contain between 4% and 7% ginsenosides. Taking 200 to 400 milligrams daily for up to eight weeks is considered safe.

 Watch out

No herbal supplement or preparation is perfect. Despite ginseng's track record of health benefits, occasionally people experience side effects like insomnia, nervousness, skin reactions, or digestive problems. Ask your doctor before starting a ginseng supplement because it may interact with certain medications like warfarin, aspirin, heparin, and antidepressants.

And while ginseng supplements are generally considered safe, lab tests have shown that some products don't contain the advertised amounts of helpful compounds. Put on your super sleuth hat to find the best products. Use sites like *ConsumerLab.com* or *labdoor.com* for objective evaluations of supplement purity.

Call on ginseng to curb high cholesterol

Nearly 94 million Americans have high cholesterol levels. That's bad news. This waxy, fatty substance that builds up in blood vessels is a major risk factor for stroke and heart disease. To make matters worse, many people don't even realize they have high cholesterol because this condition has no symptoms. The good news? Recent research suggests that ginseng could help lower cholesterol levels.

In a small study published in *Nutrients*, Korean researchers recruited 68 women with high cholesterol and sorted them into two groups. Half of the volunteers received 2 grams of Korean red ginseng extract every day, while the other half received a placebo. After four weeks, researchers examined the volunteer's blood and found that the ginseng group had lower cholesterol levels than the people who took the placebo.

If you're interested in trying it yourself, make sure to track down the right kind of ginseng. Siberian and American ginseng are different from Korean ginseng, and don't have all the same health benefits.

Underrated berries steal the spotlight with blood sugar benefits

Most ginseng supplements on store shelves are made from the root. But that doesn't mean the rest of the plant is useless. Say hello to ginseng berries.

These berries don't have a ton of research to their name, but they're packed with healthy compounds, like those ginsenosides that have made ginseng root so popular. Though hard to find, you might spot ginseng berry juice concentrate in specialty stores or online. Expect a neutral, slightly tart taste. Why go to the trouble? Better blood sugar, that's why.

Korean researchers conducted a study to put this herbal remedy to the test. They divided 63 people into two groups. Some received a placebo, while the others took an extract made from Korean ginseng berries. After 12 weeks, the people who took ginseng saw bigger decreases in their fasting blood sugar compared to the people who got the placebo.

The authors of this study aren't exactly sure why these berries might help people manage their blood sugar, but they have a few theories based on past research. Animal studies show that ginseng berry extract may increase insulin sensitivity, which makes it easier for your body to break down and use sugars.

Rosemary

Restore and revive — natural solutions for your head and hair woes

Rosemary is traditionally used to kill bacteria and fungi plus treat poor circulation. Maybe that's why this terrific-smelling essential oil is a natural when it comes to scalp and hair problems.

Soothe your dry, itchy head. Skip those smelly medicated shampoos and start feeling clean and refreshed with an easy herbal treatment.

Blend together 4 tablespoons of olive oil with 4 tablespoons of honey, and mix in 3 drops of rosemary essential oil. Heat the mixture in a double boiler until it's warm — not hot. Then massage into your damp hair and scalp. Let it sit for 30 minutes before washing out.

Get thicker, fuller hair. If it seems you have more hair in your comb than on your head, it may be time for an essential oil intervention.

For six months, men suffering from androgenetic alopecia, the most common type of hair loss, applied less than an ounce of either rosemary oil lotion or 2% topical minoxidil to their scalp every day. At the end of the study, rosemary oil proved to be just as effective at slowing hair loss and increasing hair growth as minoxidil. In addition, the men in the rosemary group had fewer side effects. Wouldn't you rather use a drug-free therapy?

Just avoid getting any essential oil in your eyes, and never apply rosemary oil directly to your skin. Always dilute it with a carrier oil like coconut, jojoba, grapeseed, or rosehip.

✕ Kitchen hacks

Change the flavor of olive oil by infusing it with dried herbs and spices. Simply add the dried sprigs, leaves, seeds, or peel directly to a bottle of olive oil, cap it tightly, and store in a cool, dark place. The oil will begin to pick up flavor within a few weeks. Try rosemary, red pepper flakes, basil, dill, dried garlic, or cumin.

Infusing works best with dried herbs and spices. Fresh ones, even garlic and citrus peel, contain enough water to grow dangerous bacteria like the one that causes botulism. If you really want to use fresh herbs from your garden, do so wisely. Mix your fresh ingredients, add to the olive oil, and keep refrigerated. Use the oil within one week.

Sharpen your mind with some help from this common herb

Ancient Greek students used to prepare for their exams by chowing down on rosemary and weaving this Mediterranean herb into garlands that they could wear while they studied. The reason? They thought this herb could help sharpen their memories. Now, modern researchers have evidence to suggest there's some truth behind these practices. New studies show that rosemary can help boost your brainpower in two surprising ways.

Sprinkle this savory herb onto your plate to stay sharp for years to come. In a small study, researchers recruited seniors and gave them either rosemary or a placebo before putting their memories to the test. The study revealed that, after taking about 1/2 teaspoon of dried rosemary, volunteers were able to recall memories faster than when they took a placebo. However, don't go overboard. The researchers found that higher doses of rosemary actually impaired the volunteers' memories.

If you're looking for interesting ways to get more rosemary in your meals, you can always add it to spice rubs for meat and poultry, or sprinkle a dash of dried rosemary in stews and soups. You can also mix it into Greek yogurt and use in place of mayo in a sandwich or potato salad.

Need to jog your memory? Take a whiff of rosemary. You don't need to eat rosemary to get brain-boosting benefits. A small study presented at a British Psychological Society conference revealed that the scent of this herb may improve people's memory.

"In this study we focused on prospective memory, which involves the ability to remember events that will occur in the future and to remember to complete tasks at particular times," says study co-author Mark Moss, Ph.D. "For example when someone needs to remember to post a birthday card or to take medication at a particular time."

Scientists divided 66 people into two groups. Some were placed in a room that was scented with rosemary essential oil, while the others sat in a room with no scent. Then they were given the memory test. Amazingly, the people in the rosemary-scented room performed better.

> For cooking purposes, cut the top 2 to 3 inches of sprigs from established rosemary plants. Don't cut too close to the plant. You need to leave some green leaves so the plant will continue to produce. If you are planning to dry the rosemary, don't harvest until the plant starts to bloom.

3 creative ways to use up your extra herbs

Gardeners love growing rosemary bushes because they are easy to care for, are naturally bug-resistant, and can thrive for years and years. But sometimes you're left with way more rosemary than you could ever eat. Here are a few ways to use it around the house.

- **Keep bugs at bay.** Creepy crawlies hate the powerful scent that comes off this herb, so planting a few rosemary shrubs around your patio or garden can help repel pests. If you want to bring this protection indoors, create a simple spray by boiling 2 cups of water with 1/2 cup of dried rosemary for 30 minutes. Strain out the herbs after the water cools and spritz it around the house to fend off insects.

- **Liven up your homemade cleaner.** Cleaning your kitchen with vinegar? Add in a few sprigs of dried rosemary and some lemon peel to freshen the scent before you use it.

- **Whip up an air freshener.** Simmer a saucepan of water on the stove, and add in a few slices of lemon, fresh or dried rosemary, a cinnamon stick, and a dash of vanilla extract. You can experiment with different herbs, spices, and fruits depending on the season.

 Bright idea

Make delicious herb bombs using ice cube trays, and enjoy your fresh herbs all year long. Here's what you'll need.

- fresh herbs such as rosemary, basil, oregano, and thyme

- olive oil

- silicone ice cube tray

Wash and pat herbs dry, and chop them into small pieces. Pack the herbs into the ice cube molds. Fill about three-quarters full. Pour oil on top, and use a fork to press the herbs into the mold.

Cover the tray with plastic wrap, and put it in the freezer for several hours or until solid. Pop the fat bombs out and place them in a freezer-proof container.

When ready to use in your favorite dish, grab a couple of bombs and drop them in to add a burst of flavor.

Sage

2 surprising ways this plant keeps you in tiptop shape

Folks have been using sage for hundreds of years to boost their brainpower. In fact, the well-known herbalist John Gerard wrote in 1597 that sage was "singularly good for the head and brain and quickeneth the nerves and memory." Centuries later, modern researchers say his guidance still holds true.

Beef up your brain with this sage advice. In a small study published in *Nutrients*, researchers from the United Kingdom pitted sage against a placebo to see if this plant could really improve people's memory. Volunteers were split into two groups and given either a daily placebo or a capsule containing 600 milligrams of sage extracts over four weeks.

At the beginning and end of the study, the volunteers completed a series of exams designed to test their memories. Lo and behold, the researchers discovered that the sage group saw improvements in their working memory after both their first and last dose. That's the kind of short-term recall you need for day-to-day tasks. The exact reason for this herb's memory-boosting benefits aren't clear, but past research on sage oil suggests that its compounds may have powerful antioxidant and anti-inflammatory effects.

Call on this herb to destress. Feel nervous and edgy sometimes? If that's the case, you might want to take a deep whiff of earthy sage. It's a great choice if you want to soothe your anxiety.

That's according to a small study of women who were undergoing a medical test. Can you guess what happened after they inhaled sage essential oil? Their blood pressure, respiration, and pulse rates — which rise under stressful conditions — all dropped. Not a bad way to relax, huh?

 Bright idea

Have some extra sage leaves lying around? Try these creative ways to use this herb.

- Repel insects the natural way. You can leave a few dried sage leaves scattered around your linens or kitchen to help keep moths and other pests at bay. Adding a handful of the leaves to an outdoor fire will also keep bugs away.

- Whip up a homemade all-purpose cleaner. Combine crushed sage leaves, 1/2 cup of warm water, 1/2 cup of white vinegar, 1/4 cup of isopropyl alcohol, and a drop of dish soap in a spray bottle. Shake it vigorously and use it to wipe clean dirty countertops and floors.

- Sore muscles? Put a muslin bag full of sage leaves into a bathtub and add hot water. Some swear that soaking in water infused with these leaves can help relieve aches and pain.

Stop plaque in its tracks with this aromatic herb

Keeping your pearly whites clean and healthy is about more than maintaining a sparkling smile. Poor dental health, including uncontrolled oral bacteria and gum inflammation, has been linked to heart problems, Alzheimer's disease, and dementia. So if you want to protect your entire body, you'll appreciate a little extra help keeping your mouth clean.

Aside from brushing, flossing, and taking regular trips to the dentist, you can add another layer of protection with a surprising garden staple. Research suggests that sage-based mouthwash can fend off the bacteria that causes plaque and tooth decay.

In a small study, volunteers used a mouthwash containing sage extract or a placebo rinse for 21 days. And at the end of the three weeks, the researchers found that the people who swished with the herbal solution saw significant reductions in the levels of *Streptococcus mutans* bacteria in their mouth. The folks who used the placebo didn't get the same benefits.

You may be able buy mouthwashes made with sage at your local pharmacy or order them online. However, you can also make your own by mixing a handful of fresh sage leaves with 1 cup of water and 1 teaspoon of salt. Bring the solution to a boil, strain it out, and let it cool before storing in an airtight container.

Don't let long-lasting menopause symptoms plague your golden years

Experts say that nearly 3 out of 4 women in menopause don't treat their symptoms. Even worse? These night sweats, hot flashes, and lapses in concentration can last for well over a decade. There's good news, though. You may be able to find relief in your spice cabinet.

New research shows that compounds found in sage may hold the key to soothing many of the worst menopause symptoms. Scientists recruited postmenopausal women and asked them to take a 100 milligram capsule of sage extract every day. Over the course of four weeks, the volunteers kept track of how severe their concentration problems, sleep troubles, fatigue, and hot flashes were. At the end of the study, the researchers found that sage helped ease these symptoms.

More study is needed to determine just how much sage you would need to eat to see these same benefits. In the meantime, you can enjoy this herb in pasta sauces, sprinkled on roast meat or vegetables, or in your favorite soups.

Turmeric

3 ways this golden spice hones your mind

Turmeric is all the rage these days. You can find this simple spice in supplements, teas, and even juices at grocery stores across the country. And there's a good reason for that — research shows turmeric offers up serious brain-boosting benefits.

Pile on the turmeric to ward off Alzheimer's. Want to win the war against Alzheimer's disease (AD)? Call on a spice you may have in your pantry right now. Turmeric — the golden spice that gives curries their distinct yellow color — is prized for its antioxidant and anti-inflammatory powers. And experts think this spice may keep your mind in tiptop shape, too.

Research suggests curcumin — the main active ingredient in turmeric — prevents the formation and growth of beta-amyloid plaques found in the brains of people with AD. Even better? Scientists have found that it may be even more successful at stopping new plaques from forming in your brain than the nonsteroidal anti-inflammatory drugs ibuprofen and naproxen.

Spice up your memory with curcumin. Your memory may not work as well as it used to. But this spice may bring it back to fighting form.

A recent study in the *American Journal of Geriatric Psychiatry* found that curcumin supplements helped improve the memories in seniors with mild cognitive impairment. Forty older adults with this condition had their cognitive abilities assessed and then were asked to take either 90 milligrams (mg) of curcumin twice a day or a placebo.

At the end of the 18-month study, the researchers retested the seniors. They found that, compared with the control group, those taking curcumin had significant improvements in their ability to remember things and pay attention. The authors think curcumin helps reduce inflammation in the brain associated with memory problems.

Want to try it yourself? You'd have to eat about 2 teaspoons of turmeric a day to get the same amount of curcumin. If you want to take a supplement instead, talk to your doctor to see if that could work for you.

Feeling blue? Improve your mood naturally. Don't let depression dog your golden years. Research from the *Journal of Affective Disorders* says turmeric may lift your spirits. In a small study, scientists asked people with severe depression to take either 500 mg of curcumin supplements twice a day or a placebo.

At the end of eight weeks, the researchers found that curcumin was a lot more effective than the placebo in improving symptoms of depression. They say this compound may help fight off the high levels of inflammation often found in people with severe depression.

 Bright idea

Coloring eggs isn't just for Easter. It's also a good way to tell hard-boiled eggs from raw ones. You don't even need to buy food coloring to tint your eggs. These foods make great natural dyes. Just add them to a mixture of vinegar and water.

Beet juice turns your eggs pink while red cabbage turns them blue. For yellow, choose turmeric. For red, try paprika. Spinach works for green, and blueberries work for purple. Brewed coffee will turn your eggs brown.

Experiment with nature's rainbow. You'll find plenty of colorful foods right in your own kitchen.

End inflammation-related issues with a heaping helping of turmeric

When your body detects germs or damaged tissue, your immune system sends inflammatory cells to trap bacteria and kick-start the healing process. And that's a good thing. But other times, your body continues to dispatch these cells long after the danger has passed.

It's called chronic inflammation, and it's been linked to several health conditions, including depression. So if you want to boost your mood and get relief, try enlisting the help of the powerful anti-inflammatory food turmeric.

Control blood sugar with this golden spice. Long-term inflammation can interfere with insulin's ability to tell your cells to absorb the glucose they need. This leads to high blood sugar, which along with insulin resistance, can cause even more inflammation. Left untreated, this vicious cycle often develops into type 2 diabetes.

That's where turmeric comes in. Research shows that the main compound in turmeric — curcumin — helps regulate the body's inflammatory response and lowers insulin resistance. In fact, one study found that people who took curcumin for nine months didn't develop type 2 diabetes after being diagnosed with high blood sugar. That's astonishing when you consider that 16% of the placebo group did.

Want to melt belly fat away? Eating turmeric helps shed extra pounds. Experts say that carrying around extra weight can cause inflammation to spike throughout your body. This can lead to a host of health problems, including high blood pressure.

But here's the good news. Losing the excess weight eases the related inflammation. And the colorful spice turmeric may just help you do that. A review of 21 studies found that people who took curcumin experienced drops in both their weight and waist size. A possible reason why? Curcumin increases the amount of adiponectin in the blood. This hormone helps regulate fat and glucose metabolism.

Relieve arthritis pain without drugs. Is your arthritis pain flaring up? You may want to pop a pill to ease the pain. But long-term use of nonsteroidal anti-inflammatory drugs — such as ibuprofen — can have dangerous side effects, including an increased risk of peptic ulcer. Fortunately, you can get natural relief from turmeric.

One study found that curcumin was just as effective at treating arthritis pain and stiffness as an over-the-counter drug thanks to it's powerful anti-inflammatory effects. People in this study took 500 milligrams of curcumin three times a day for a month. You can find curcumin supplements online or at some grocery stores.

 Kitchen hacks

Remember stirring cocoa powder into milk for a yummy after-school treat? If you loved drinking chocolate milk, you might want to try this grown-up version. Golden milk, made by mixing turmeric and other spices into your drink, is a tasty treat that can help keep you healthy.

- Bring 1 cup of milk or nondairy milk to a simmer in a small saucepan.

- Whisk in 1/2 teaspoon of ground turmeric. You can add a bit more if you want a stronger flavor. Or if it tastes too intense, dial the turmeric back a bit.

- Stir in a few of your favorite spices. Try mixing in a dash of cinnamon, grated fresh ginger, whole cardamon pods, or even a pinch of black pepper. Want it sweet? Try adding a spoonful of honey.

- Strain out any solids and give it a final stir to combine. Serve warm or chill in the fridge.

Kiss cancer goodbye with this super spice

Turmeric has been used as a medicinal spice for over 4,500 years. And it's easy to see why. Curcumin, the naturally-occuring phytochemical in turmeric, may help prevent cancer all over the body. Read on for the wonders it can do.

Colon. Curcumin keeps blood vessels from providing oxygen and nutrients to cancer cells and might also charge up vitamin D in the colon, where experts say it acts as a cancer-fighting agent.

Breast. Research published in the journal *Breast Cancer Research and Treatment* says curcumin may prevent breast cancer cells from forming, growing, and spreading. And a review of several studies published in *Integrative Biology* says curcumin shows promise as a way to prevent breast cancer. But if you already have breast cancer, talk with your doctor. Some studies suggest that curcumin interferes with cyclophosphamide, a chemotherapy drug.

Prostate. This cancer takes several years to kick into full gear and is often related to a high-fat diet, lack of exercise — and inflammation. But curcumin seems to halt the inflammation that can lead to prostate cancer.

Brain. Experts from MD Anderson Cancer Center say curcumin prevents brain cancer cells from growing and spreading, and encourages the death of cancer cells.

Leukemia. When someone has leukemia, or cancer of the blood cells, their bone marrow produces abnormal white blood cells. Called leukemia cells, they grow fast and crowd out normal blood cells. Scientists think curcumin triggers an excessive production of reactive oxygen species — molecules that promote leukemia cell death.

Melanoma. This skin cancer is the deadliest of all skin cancers. But a recent German study suggests that curcumin inhibits the growth of melanoma cancer cells.

Pancreas. Cook curcumin with olive oil for a tasty way to block pancreatic cancer. A study published in the journal *Nutrition and Cancer* proposes that the combination of curcumin and omega-3 fatty acids may prevent, battle, and kill pancreatic cancer cells.

Head and neck. Scientists believe the golden spice shuts down the communication between cells that trigger cancer cell growth. It also lowers the number of pro-inflammatory cytokines — substances that promote inflammation and cancer growth. Many experts suggest taking curcumin as a supplement, because you can't get the amount you need to fight head and neck cancer from spicing up your food.

 Kitchen hacks

Have a recipe calling for turmeric? Don't run for the spice rack just yet. A fresher option may be sitting right next to its knobby-jointed cousin — ginger root — in the produce aisle.

At first glance, turmeric root may not look like much. But under its dull brown peel lies bright orange flesh eager to add a peppery edge to your next meal.

When preparing fresh turmeric, wear kitchen gloves to avoid getting orange-yellow stains on your fingers. Scrape off the paper-thin peel with a spoon. Grate the root into marinades, dips, eggs, smoothies, and stir-fries. Or for a bit of added crunch, cut turmeric into thin matchsticks for salads.

As a general rule, 1 tablespoon of freshly grated turmeric is equal to 1 teaspoon of the ground spice.

Store fresh turmeric in an airtight container in the fridge for up to two weeks.

Index

A

Acid reflux. *See* Heartburn
Acne 8
Adaptogen 345
Adenosine 305
Age-related macular degeneration
  (AMD)
  apricots for 117
  berries for 134
  grapes for 157-158
  oats for 180-181
  olive oil for 41-42
  oysters for 280-281
  peppers for 96
  salmon for 290
  spinach for 82
Air freshener 342, 351
Allergens 223, 309
Allicin 88-89
Aloe vera 2-6
Aloin 3
Alpha-linolenic acid (ALA)
  for heart 263
  good sources of 258, 263, 308
Alternative sweeteners 29-30
Alzheimer's disease
  berries for 131
  coffee for 302-303
  kombucha for 238

MIND diet for 35-36
  peppers for 93
  sweet potatoes for 99
  turmeric for 355
Amaranth 191
Androgenetic alopecia 348
Anise 334-335
Anthocyanins
  for Alzheimer's disease 131
  for diabetes 113, 154
  for heart disease 61
  for high blood pressure 61
  for high cholesterol 62
  for Parkinson's disease 131
  good sources of 101
Anxiety. *See* Stress
Apples 110-114
Apricots 115-118
Arsenic 174-175
Arthritis. *See* Joint pain
Arugula 79-80
Aspartame 29
Aspirin 7-9
Avocados 119-124

B

Bad breath
  fennel seeds for 262
  yogurt for 252

Baking powder, substitute for 18
Baking soda 10-17
Bananas 125-128
Barley 168-172
Beans 202-207
Beets 52-54
Berries 129-135
Beta carotene, good sources of 93,
    98-99, 103, 117, 158
Beta glucans
    for chronic inflammation 313
    for diabetes 168-169, 179, 313
    for heart disease 168, 179
    for high cholesterol 34
    for immune system 34
    good sources of 33-34, 168, 179,
        313
Bladder cancer 286
Blood clots
    aspirin for 8
    garlic for 72
    sorghum for 193
    thrombotic stroke and 284-285
    walnuts for 275
Blood sugar control. *See* Diabetes
Bok choy 80
Bone loss. *See* Osteoporosis
Boron 164-165
Brain cancer 359
Breast cancer
    broccoli for 56
    cantaloupe for 162-163
    olive oil for 37
    soy supplements and 226
    tomatoes for 106
    turmeric for 359
    walnuts for 276
    yogurt for 255-256

Broccoli 55-59
Brown rice 173-175
Brown sugar, substitute for 18
Bug bites
    baking soda for 13
    bananas for 128
    cinnamon for 338

C

Cabbage 60-62
Caffeine
    diabetes and 301
    for Alzheimer's disease 303
    for energy 305
    for Parkinson's disease 304
    good sources of 304
    in tea 324
    sleep and 305
Calcium oxalate 81
Cancer. *See Also* Specific cancers
    broccoli for 56, 59
    citrus for 145
    flaxseeds for 265
    kombucha for 238-239
    oats for 180
    olive oil for 36-37
    onions for 88-89
    quinoa for 186
    raw oysters and 282
    walnuts for 275
Canker sores
    cinnamon and 339
    honey for 28
Capsaicin
    for Alzheimer's disease 93
    for heart disease 92-93

for high cholesterol 91-92
for joint pain 90
for psoriasis 90
for sore muscles 90
for weight loss 90-91
Carpet stains 11
Cataracts
  apricots for 117
  peppers for 95
  spinach for 82
Cauliflower 63-66
Cavities
  aloe vera for 5
  cloves for 341-342
  fennel seeds for 262
  honey for 27
  sage for 354
Celiac disease
  barley and 170
  oats and 176
  sorghum and 194
Chard 80
Chemicals, in tap water 329
Cherries 137-141
Chia seeds 258-260
Chickpeas 209-213
Chlorogenic acid 301
Chocolate 19-24
Cholesterol. *See* High cholesterol
Choline 65-66
Chronic inflammation
  apricots for 118
  oat milk for 313
  oysters for 282-283
  salmon for 289-290
  turmeric for 357
  walnuts for 277-278

Cinnamon 336-339
Citrus 142-148
Cleaning
  baking soda for 10-12
  cloves for 342
  lemon juice for 146
  rice for 174
  rosemary for 351
  sage for 353
Clogged drains, clearing 13
Cloves 340-342
Cocoa, for peripheral artery disease
  (PAD) 23-24
Coenzyme Q10 298
Coffee 300-305
Coffee, substitute for 213
Cognitive function
  apples for 114
  beets for 53
  berries for 132-133
  cauliflower for 65-66
  cherry juice for 137-138
  chocolate for 19
  flaxseeds for 266
  garlic for 75
  greens for 78-79
  nutritional yeast for 31
  olive oil for 35
  onions for 88
  pecans for 267-268
  prunes for 164
  rosemary for 349-350
  sage for 352
  salmon for 289
  sardines for 294-295
  sauerkraut for 248
  turmeric for 355-356
  walnuts for 276

Cognitive function *(continued)*
  water for 325-326
  yogurt for 251
Colorectal cancer
  cabbage for 60-61
  garlic for 74
  raspberries for 129
  spinach for 82
  sugar-sweetened beverages and 29
  turmeric for 359
  walnuts for 276
  wheat bran for 197-198
  yogurt for 254-255
Common cold
  honey for 26-27
  nutritional yeast for 34
Constipation
  cabbage for 60
  figs for 150-151
  popcorn for 183
  prunes for 165-166
  water for 329-330
  wheat bran for 197
Cooking tips
  for barley 171
  for beet greens 54
  for broccoli 57
  for brown rice 174-175
  for cauliflower 64
  for chia seeds 260
  for cloves 341
  for dried beans 17, 205
  for eggplant 69
  for eggs 49-50
  for garlic 71
  for grapes 158
  for green beans 49
  for kimchi 236-237

  for kombucha 239
  for lentils 216
  for marinating 293
  for oats 178
  for onions 89
  for pasta 49, 332
  for peanut butter 223
  for peanut oil 223
  for pecans 268
  for peppers 91, 96
  for pie crust 49
  for popcorn 184
  for potatoes 100, 102
  for quinoa 186, 187-188
  for red cabbage 62
  for rosemary 350
  for salmon 288, 291
  for sardines 296
  for sesame oil 272
  for sesame seeds 271
  for sorghum 195
  for spinach 81
  for sweet potato leaves 98
  for yogurt 252
  to mask bitterness 6, 24
  to reduce acidity 17, 302
  to tenderize meat 17
Copper 190, 269-270
Cornstarch 11
Cortisol 20
Cream of tartar, substitute for 18
Creamer, substitute for 305
Curcumin
  for Alzheimer's disease 355
  for chronic inflammation 357
  for cognitive function 355-356
  for depression 356
  for diabetes 357

for joint pain 358
for weight loss 357-358

D

DASH diet 78
Deodorant 13
Depression
  anise for 334
  chocolate for 20
  coffee for 304-305
  kombucha for 238
  nutritional yeast for 32
  sauerkraut for 247-248
  soybeans for 227
  turmeric for 356
Diabetes
  aloe vera for 4
  apples for 112-113
  barley for 168-169
  beans for 206
  berries for 129-130
  brown rice for 173
  caffeine and 301
  cinnamon tea for 319
  cloves for 340
  coffee for 301
  eggplant for 68
  ginseng berries for 347
  grapefruit for 143-144
  grapes for 154
  kimchi for 234
  lentils for 215-216
  oat milk for 313
  oats for 179
  peanuts for 220-221
  pecans for 269

peppers for 90
raw oysters and 282
sesame oil for 273
sorghum for 195-196
turmeric for 357
vinegar for 45
Dish soap
  for cleaning carpets 11
  for killing weeds 48
  for pest control 28

E

E. coli 337
Eggplant 67-69
Eggs, substitute for 18, 212, 213,
  260
Equol 227
Exotic fruits 152-153

F

Farro 191
Fennel seeds 261-262
Fermentation 250
Fiber
  for colorectal cancer 60-61
  for constipation 60, 150-151
  for diabetes 68
  for high cholesterol 62, 68, 141
  for weight loss 67-68, 87, 110-111
  good sources of 110-111, 116,
    119-120, 150, 166, 204-205,
    216, 247
  juicing and 76
  recommended intake 62, 330

Fibromyalgia, olive oil for 42
Figs 149-151
Flaxseeds 263-266
Flour
    barley 169
    chickpea 213
    peanut 222
    quinoa 186
    sorghum 194
FODMAP sensitivity
    cauliflower and 66
    plant milks for 307
    prebiotics and 233
Folate
    for cognitive function 78-79
    good sources of 79, 84, 210
    recommended intake 84
Food coloring, substitute for 356
Food poisoning 293, 337
Food substitutions 18
    beans 208
    for coffee 213
    for creamer 305
    for eggs 212, 213, 260
    for ground beef 218
    for mayonnaise 252
    for molasses 196
    for salt 95
    for sugar 29-30
    for white rice 171-172, 173,
        195-196
Foot problems
    baking soda for 13
    olive oil for 40

G

Gardening tips
    for avoiding pests 92
    for killing weeds 48
    for storing tomato seeds 108
    with garlic 73
Garlic 70-75
Gas
    anise tea for 334-335
    caraway seeds for 335
    cauliflower and 66
    chamomile tea for 335
    cinnamon for 338
    fennel seeds for 262, 335
    peppermint leaves for 335
    prebiotics and 233
    vinegar and 46
    wheat bran and 199
Gastroesophageal reflux disease
    (GERD). See Heartburn
Gingivitis. See Gum disease
Ginseng 345-347
Gout. See Joint pain
Grapes 154-158
Grass allergies, sorghum and 194
Greens 78-85
    beet greens 53-54
Grilling 292-293
Ground beef, substitute for 218
Gum disease
    aloe vera for 6
    baking soda for 14-15
    honey for 27

H

H. pylori 56, 88
Hair care
  baking soda for 12
  lentils for 215
  oats for 181
  olive oil for 40
  rosemary oil for 348
Hair loss 348
Hashimoto's disease 4
HDL cholesterol. *See* High
  cholesterol
Head and neck cancer 360
Headaches
  aspirin for 9
  fermented foods and 249
  salmon for 289-290
  water for 331-332
Heart disease
  apples for 112
  aspirin for 8
  barley for 168
  beans for 206
  blueberries for 130
  broccoli for 55-56
  cherries for 141
  chocolate for 21-22
  citrus for 142-143
  coffee for 300
  collard greens for 83-84
  flax milk for 308-309
  flaxseeds for 263
  kefir for 230-231
  lentils for 214-215
  oats for 179
  olive oil for 38
  oysters for 283

  peanuts for 221
  peppers for 92-93
  quinoa for 186
  red cabbage for 61
  sardines for 297
  sesame seeds for 273
  sorghum for 193
  tea for 318-319
  tofu for 224
  walnuts for 274
Heartburn
  aloe vera for 4
  baking soda for 17
  peppermint tea and 322
  vinegar and 44
Hemorrhagic stroke. *See* Stroke
Hemorrhoids, wheat bran for 197
Hesperidin 145, 148
High blood pressure
  apricots for 116
  bananas for 128
  beets for 52-53
  cherry juice for 141
  cinnamon for 336-337
  eggplant for 68
  garlic 71
  miso for 241
  olive oil for 38-39
  orange juice for 148
  red cabbage for 61
  sardines for 296-297
  sesame seeds for 273
  skim milk for 315
  sorghum for 193
  tea for 318-319
  walnuts for 274-275
  water for 328-329
  watermelon for 160

High blood pressure *(continued)*
  wheat bran for 199
  yogurt for 251-252
High cholesterol
  apples for 112
  apricots for 116
  avocados for 121
  barley for 168
  black tea for 319
  broccoli for 55, 59
  cherry juice for 141
  chia seeds for 258
  cinnamon for 336
  eggplant for 68
  flaxseeds for 308
  garlic for 70-71
  ginseng for 346-347
  honey for 25
  kefir for 230
  nutritional yeast for 34
  oats for 179
  pecans for 268
  peppers for 91-92
  red cabbage for 62
  red grapes for 155
  skim milk for 315-316
  soy milk for 309
  spinach for 82-83
  vinegar for 44
Honey 25-28
  substitute for 18
Hummus 211-212
Hypertension. *See* High blood
  pressure
Hypothyroidism 4

Immune system
  bananas for 125
  broccoli for 56
  ginseng for 345
  goji berries for 133
  lentils for 215
  nutritional yeast for 34
  peppers for 96
  raw oysters and 282
  sauerkraut for 248-249
  tomatoes for 103
Indigestion
  coffee and 302
  fennel seeds for 262
  peppermint tea for 322
Inflammatory bowel disease (IBD)
  322
Insomnia 126
Insulin resistance. *See* Diabetes
Inulin 86-87
Iron
  for fighting fatigue 115, 170
  for healthy blood 281, 311-312
  for heart health 214-215
  for immune system 215
  for RLS 214
  for thinning hair 215
  good sources of 80, 170, 190,
    191, 214, 281, 312
Irritable bowel syndrome (IBS)
  cauliflower and 66
  fennel seeds for 262
  figs for 151
  plant milks for 307
  sauerkraut for 245

J

Jackfruit 152
Joint pain
   apples for 111
   bitter melon for 163
   broccoli for 57-58
   cabbage for 62
   cherries for 138-139
   cherry juice for 139-140
   flaxseeds for 264-265
   garlic for 72
   sesame seeds for 271
   turmeric for 358
   vinegar for 50
   water for 330-331
   yogurt for 256
Juicing 76-77
   beets 54

K

Kaempferol 59, 185
Kefir 230-232
Khorasan wheat 192
Kidney cancer
   bananas for 127-128
   tomatoes for 106
Kidney disease
   baking soda for 15-16
   vinegar and 44
Kidney stones
   honeydew melon for 161-162
   skim milk for 314
   soy milk for 225
   water for 327
Kimchi 234-237

Kombucha 238-240

L

Lactose intolerance 306-307
Lard, substitute for 18
Latex 3, 5, 127
LDL cholesterol. *See* High
   cholesterol
Lemon juice, substitute for 18
Lentils 214-218
Leukemia 359
Lignans
   for cancer 265
   for cognitive function 266
   for weight control 266
Liver cancer, tomatoes for 107
Liver disease, raw oysters and 282
Lung cancer, tomatoes for 106-107
Lutein
   for cognitive function 79
   for eyes 59, 82, 96, 123-124
   good sources of 79, 124
Lychees 152

M

Magnesium
   for diabetes 303
   for heart 54
   for immune system 54
   for insomnia 126
   for joint pain 265
   for mood 82
   good sources of 82, 126, 149,
      159-160, 175, 190, 194
   recommended intake 265

Manganese
  for bones 54, 175
  for energy production 170
  good sources of 170, 175, 269
Mangoes 153
Marinating 293
Mattress, cleaning 11
Mayonnaise, substitute for 18, 252
Medication risks
  anise and 334
  aspirin and 7-8, 9
  cauliflower and 66
  cloves and 340
  garlic and 72
  ginseng and 346
  grapefruit and 144
  nonsteroidal anti-inflammatory
    drugs 139, 358
  nutritional yeast and 34
  star fruit and 153
  vinegar and 45
  vitamin K and 157
Mediterranean diet
  for AMD 41
  for NAFLD 217-218
Melanoma 359
Melatonin 138
Melons 159-163
Menopause symptoms
  fennel seeds for 261
  sage for 354
Mercury 281, 285, 288
Metabolic syndrome
  beans for 206-207
  quinoa for 189
  sweet potatoes for 99
Migraines. *See* Headaches

Milk, substitute for 18
Miso 241-244
Molasses, substitute for 196
Monosodium glutamate (MSG) 228
Monounsaturated fatty acids
  (MUFAs)
  for high blood pressure 221
  for high cholesterol 221
  for weight loss 40
  good sources of 40, 124, 221, 267
Mouthwash
  aloe vera 6
  honey 27-28
  sage 354
Muscle weakness. *See* Sarcopenia
Mustard greens 80

N

Natto 244
Nitrates 52-53
Nonalcoholic fatty liver disease
  (NAFLD) 217-218
Nutmeg, substitute for 18
Nutritional yeast 31-34

O

Oats 176-181
Odor control
  baking soda for 11, 13
  garlic and 75
  rosemary for 351
  vinegar and 47
Olive oil 35-42
Omega-3 fatty acids

for AMD 290
for chronic inflammation 282-283
for headaches 289-290
for heart disease 297
for high blood pressure 296-297
for memory loss 289, 294-295
for stroke 297
good sources of 274, 283, 284, 294
Onions 86-89
Organic produce 97
Osteoporosis
chia seeds for 258-259
figs for 149-150
garlic for 73
grapes for 156-157
kimchi for 236
olive oil for 39-40
prunes for 164-165
skim milk for 316-317
spinach for 81
sweet potatoes for 99
tea for 320-321
yogurt for 251
Oysters 280-283

P

Pancreatic cancer 360
Papaya 153
Parkinson's disease
berries for 131-132
coffee for 303-304
Passion fruit 153
Peanuts 220-223
Pecans 267-270
Peppers 90-96

Periodontal disease. *See* Gum disease
Peripheral artery disease (PAD),
cocoa for 23-24
Pest control
cayenne pepper for 92
cinnamon for 338
cloves for 342
garlic for 73
honey for 28
rosemary for 351
sage for 353
vinegar for 48
walnuts for 277
Phosphorus
for bones 190
for teeth 190
good sources of 190, 310-311
Phylloquinone 84-85
Plant milks 306-313
Polyunsaturated fatty acids
(PUFAs)
for high blood pressure 221
for high cholesterol 221
for joint pain 264-265
good sources of 221, 264, 278
Popcorn 182-184
Potassium
for bones 54
for heart 100-101
for high blood pressure 54, 61
good sources of 80, 98, 100-101
Potatoes 98-102
Prebiotics
good sources of 233
in cabbage 60
in onions 86
shopping for 233

Probiotics
  for breast cancer 255-256
  for colon cancer 254-255
  for dementia 248
  for depression 247-248
  for diabetes 234
  for heart disease 230-231
  for high cholesterol 230
  for IBS 245
  for immune system 249
  for ulcerative colitis 245-246
  for weight control 234-235,
    246-247
  supplements 250
Prostate cancer
  tomatoes for 106
  turmeric for 359
Protein
  good sources of 188, 203, 252,
    260, 309, 316
  recommended intake 309
Prunes 164-166
Psoriasis
  aspirin for 8
  bananas for 128
  capsaicin for 90
Purines 256, 331

Q

Quercetin
  for cancer 186
  for cognitive function 88
  for eyes 114
  for heart disease 186
Quinoa 185-190

R

Recipes
  almond milk 311
  barley rice 171-172
  barley tea 172
  chickpea apple salad 269-270
  chickpea coffee 213
  cinnamon tea 319, 338-339
  cold-brewed coffee 302
  fennel tea 262
  golden milk 358
  herb bombs 351
  iced tea 321
  infused olive oil 349
  infused water 326
  kefir 231-232
  marinades 293
  pecan butter 270
  pineapple spinach salad 269
  prunes 166
  roasted chickpeas 210
Reflux. *See* Heartburn
Resistant starch
  in chickpeas 210
  potatoes and 102
Resting heart rate 241-242
Restless legs syndrome (RLS) 214
Rosacea, aspirin for 8
Rosemary 348-351
Rubbing alcohol 10

S

Saccharin 30
Sage 352-354
Salmon 284-291

Salt
  headaches and 249
  how to keep fresh 174
  kimchi and 235
  recommended intake 343
  reducing intake 343-344
  substitute for 95, 343-344
Sarcopenia
  beans for 203
  cantaloupe for 162
  miso for 242-243
  nutritional yeast for 33
Sardines 294-298
Sauerkraut 245-249
Scoville heat unit 93-94
Selenium
  for cancer 202
  for memory 295
  for thyroid health 281
  good sources of 175, 202, 281,
    295
  recommended intake 295
Sesame seeds 271-273
Shopping
  for aloe vera 5
  for apples 113
  for apricots 116
  for avocados 124
  for bread 200
  for broccoli 58
  for cherries 140
  for eggplant 69
  for farro 191
  for figs 151
  for ginseng 346
  for hemp milk 312
  for honey 26
  for jackfruit 152

  for kimchi 237
  for kombucha 240
  for lox 287
  for lychees 152-153
  for mangoes 153
  for melons 161
  for miso 242, 243-244
  for nutritional yeast 32
  for oats 177-178
  for olive oil 37
  for oranges 147-148
  for organic produce 97
  for oysters 282
  for peanut butter 221
  for plant milks 312
  for powdered peanut butter 222
  for probiotic supplements 250
  for produce, in general 136
  for quinoa 187-188
  for salmon 287-288
  for sauerkraut 246
  for skim milk 317
  for smoked salmon 287
  for sorghum 194
  for sorghum syrup 196
  for teff 192
  for vinegar 46-47
  for walnut oil 278
  for yogurt 253-254
Skim milk 314-317
Skin cancer, tomatoes for 106
Skin care
  aloe vera for 2-3
  cauliflower for 65
  cocoa for 20-21
  olive oil for 40
  sesame oil for 273

Skin care (continued)
  tomatoes for 107-108
  wheat bran for 199
Skin problems
  acne 8
  aloe vera for 2
  aspirin for 8
  baking soda for 13
  bananas for 128
  citrus for 146-147
  flaxseeds for 264
  oats for 181
  psoriasis 8, 90
  rosacea 8
  rosemary oil for 348
  sesame oil for 273
  soybeans for 227-228
Sleep. See Also Insomnia
  aloe vera for 6
  chamomile tea for 323-324
  cherry juice for 138
Slow cooking 219
Soda ash 12
Sodium. See Salt
Sodium bicarbonate. See Baking
  soda
Sore muscles
  sage for 353
  tomatoes for 104
Sorghum 193-196
Sour cream, substitute for 18
Sous vide 288
Soybeans 224-228
Star fruit 153
Stevia 29
Storing food
  amaranth 191
  apricots 116

asparagus 136
bananas 136
berries 134, 136
bran 198
cherries 140
dry beans 204
figs 151
flaxseeds 266
grapes 158
greens 85
kimchi 237
miso 244
mushrooms 136
oysters 283
pecans 268
potatoes 136
produce, in general 136
prunes 166
sorghum 195
sorghum syrup 196
tomatoes 105
walnut oil 278
Stress
  chamomile tea for 323-324
  chocolate for 20
  ginseng for 345-346
  sage for 352-353
Stroke. See Also Blood clots
  aspirin and 7
  beans for 206
  cherries for 141
  chocolate for 22-23
  citrus for 142
  coffee for 300
  kimchi for 236
  salmon for 284-285
  sardines for 297
  sorghum for 193

walnuts for 274
Substitutions. *See* Food substitutions
Sucralose 30
Sugar 29-30
  in fruit juice 76-77
  plant milks and 312
  recommended intake 312
  substitute for 25-26
Sulforaphane
  for blood vessels 55
  for cancer 64
  for diabetes 63-64
  for inflammation 63
  for joint pain 57-58
Synovial fluid 330-331

T

Tannins 320, 323
Tea 318-324
Teff 192
Tempeh 244
Tomatoes 103-108
Toothpaste
  aloe vera 5
  baking soda 15
Turmeric 355-360
Turnip greens 80
Tyramine
  in fermented foods 249
  in nutritional yeast 34

U

Ulcerative colitis
  probiotics for 245-246

walnuts for 277-278
Urinary incontinence 286
Urinary tract infection 286

V

V. vulnificus 282
Vinegar 43-50
  for cleaning bathrooms 10-11
  for clogged drains 13
  for pest control 28
  for testing baking soda 16
Vitamin A
  for bones 99
  for eyes 53, 117
  for immune system 103
  good sources of 80, 133, 313
  recommended intake 99
Vitamin B12
  for depression 32
  for memory 31
  for sarcopenia 33
  good sources of 31, 280-281,
    290-291, 298
  recommended intake 33, 290-291,
    298
Vitamin B6
  for heart disease 83-84
  for immune system 125
  good sources of 84, 98, 101,
    125, 170, 202, 209
  recommended intake 84
Vitamin C
  for aging skin 53
  for cataracts 95, 117
  for heart disease 142-143

Vitamin C *(continued)*
  for immune system 103
  for strokes 142
  for weight control 143
  good sources of 56, 65, 100,
    142-143, 147, 162, 248-249
  recommended intake 117
Vitamin D
  for bladder cancer 286-287
  for urinary incontinence 286
  for urinary tract infection 286
  good sources of 286, 295, 310
  recommended intake 286
Vitamin K
  for blood clotting 59
  for bones 53
  good sources of 53, 59, 79-80,
    81, 85, 236, 244
  recommended intake 236

W

Walnuts 274-278
Water 325-332
Weight control
  apples for 110-111
  avocados for 119-121
  beans for 207
  blueberries for 135
  chia seeds for 259-260
  chocolate and 21
  cinnamon for 337
  citrus for 143
  eggplant for 67-68
  flaxseeds for 266
  honey and 25

kimchi for 234-235
oats for 176-177
olive oil for 40
onions for 87
peanuts for 220
pecans for 267
peppers for 90-91
popcorn for 182
sauerkraut for 246-247
spinach for 82
sweet potatoes for 99
tea for 318
turmeric for 357-358
vinegar for 43
watermelon for 159-160
wheat bran for 198
Wheat bran 197-200
White rice, substitute for
  barley 171-172
  brown rice 173
  millets 195-196

Y

Yogurt 251-256

Z

Zeaxanthin
  for eyes 59, 96, 124
  good sources of 124, 134
Zinc
  good sources of 179, 222,
    280-281
  recommended intake 281